Fish Oil and the Omega 3 Diet

Explaining Omega 3 fish oil and Omega 3 fatty acids including Omega 3 recipes

Ellen Vincent

Disclaimer and Terms of Use: The Author and Publisher has strived to be as accurate and complete as possible in the creation of this book, notwithstanding the fact that she does not warrant or represent at any time that the contents within are accurate due to the rapidly changing nature of science and medicine. While all attempts have been made to verify information provided in this publication, the Author and Publisher assumes no responsibility for errors, omissions, or contrary interpretation of the subject matter herein. Any perceived slights of specific persons, peoples, or organizations are unintentional. In practical advice books, like anything else in life, there are no guarantees of any results obtained. Readers are cautioned to rely on their own judgment and seek professional medical advice about their individual circumstances and to act accordingly.

First Printing, 2013

ISBN -13: 978-1492940067

ISBN -10: 1492940062

Printed in the United States of America

Dedication

For Ellen and Titus

Fish Oil and the Omega 3 Diet

Explaining Omega 3 fish oil and Omega 3 fatty acids including Omega 3 recipes

Table of Contents

Introduction

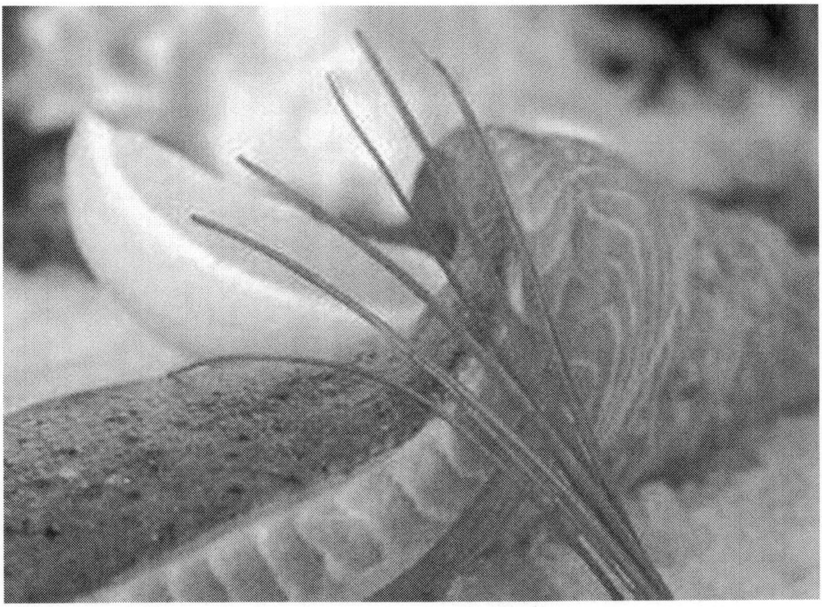

When the words oils and fats are mentioned, health-conscious individuals tend to run for cover. What they fail to realize is that there are good fats and bad fats. Complete avoidance of intake of oils and fats would actually be detrimental to health due to the fact that our bodies need them for making essential materials such as the membranes that surround every cell. Fats are also very important for the correct functioning of the nervous system. Fats and oils become a problem when the ones you eat are potentially the wrong type and eaten in the wrong amounts.

Out of the right types of oils, those providing a supply of Omega 3 fatty acids have become very popular because of the health benefits that come from consuming them. The best sources of Omega 3 are fatty fish and flaxseeds, however, the following foods are also rich in omega 3 fatty acids:

Hempseed
Perilla oil
Spirulina seaweed
Walnuts
Eggs
Chia seeds
Raddish seeds
Fresh basil
Spinach and other dark leafed greens
Dried tarragon

When choosing a food to provide your omega 3 fatty acids you need to also consider what other factors in the food might also provide benefits. Fish and flaxseeds aren't just made up of omega 3. There are many other useful substances contained within the raw food. It is possible that they enhance the observed health benefits of the omega 3. By using supplements alone you may be missing out on these extra substances and their additional properties. This is shown in the book by the comparison of fish and marine sources with flaxseeds as a source of omega 3. Obviously if you are a vegetarian then you will be concentrating on the plant sources of omega 3 rather than the fish ones.

When considering fish as a source of omega 3 fatty acids you need to realize that whereas oily fish may contain up to thirty percent oil white fish will contain much less and that it may be contained in the liver with significantly less in the flesh of the fish.

Leading authorities on the subject of nutrition are now emphasizing the benefits of including fish oil in your diet. It is generally considered to be one of the most often sought after remedies when it comes to improving physical performance, treating obesity, and improving mental focus. Clearly, the benefits of this oil can be great for your health. Wide ranged benefits that include helping your body both physically and mentally make fish oil a substance that can greatly affect your life positively in a multitude of ways.

Despite all of the concern about fat in our diet, the body does require healthy fats and oils to function. The problem is that most people are getting the wrong kinds of fats in their diet and are lacking the good, healthy fats. Besides being an energy source, healthy fats and oils are nutrients used in the production of cell membranes, as well as in several hormone like compounds called Eicosanoids.

These compounds help regulate blood pressure, heart rate, blood vessel constriction, blood clotting and the nervous system. In addition, dietary fat carries the fat soluble vitamins, which are vitamins A, D, E and K, from your food into your body. Fat also helps maintain healthy hair and skin, protects vital organs, keeps your body insulated, and provides a sense of fullness after meals so you are satiated. The human body cannot function properly without two polyunsaturated fats, which are linoleic and alphalinoleic acid. These fatty acids are found in flaxseed oil and other healthy oils. They are truly needed for normal cell structure and body function. Flaxseed may also prove useful in the nutritional management of patients with autoimmune diseases.

Getting Omega 3 from fish

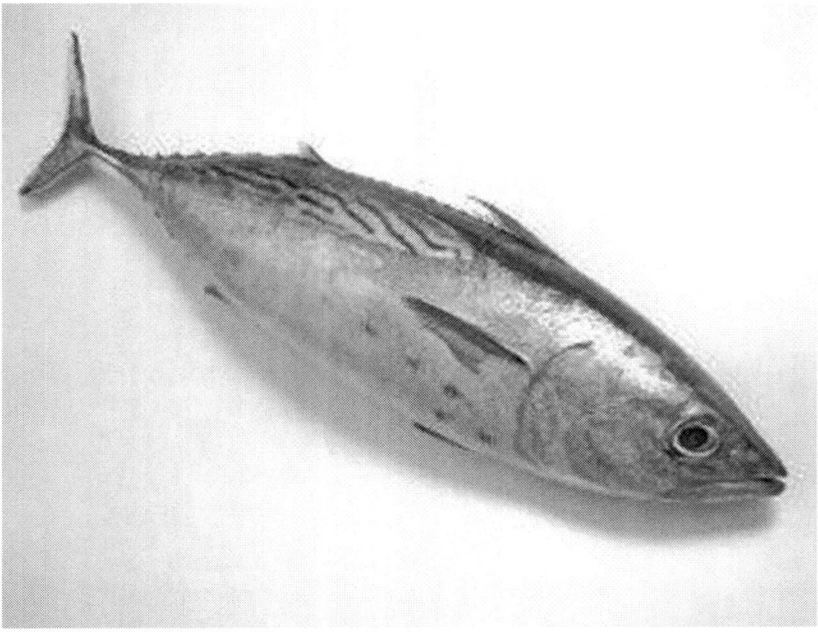

Fish obtain their Omega 3 fatty acids by eating microalgae which contain these acids. The can also get it from eating other fish that have the acids already built up from their diet on these algae. Fish that are fatty include Salmon, Tuna, smelt, anchovy, Mackerel, Lake Trout, Sardines, and Herring.

There has been a lot of hype and publicity about Omega 3 fish oils and it seems that a lot of food producers are rushing to add them to their products. There are lots of promises that have been made but what is not sometimes clear is what they actually do for the human body.

Essential fatty acids (EFA) must always be part of our daily diet because without them, we cannot manufacture important substances and we take one step closer to our deaths. Essential fatty acids are divided into two families: omega-6 EFAs and omega-3 EFAS.

Although there are only very slight differences to distinguish the two groups of essential fatty acids from each other, studies have revealed that too much intake of omega-6 EFAs can lead to inflammation, blood clotting and tumor growth. The good news, however, is that the opposite is true for omega-3 EFAs. Omega-6 EFAs can be found in vegetable oils while omega-3 EFAs can be found in fish oils among other foods.

The omega-6 EFAs found in vegetable oils includes, but is not limited to corn oil and soy oil, both of which contain high amounts of linoleic acid. Omega-3 EFAs on the other hand can also be found in marine plankton and walnut and flaxseed oils.

Omega 3 oil is a substance that can be found in the bodies of fish. Omega 3 is a type of fat that is essential for human health. Omega 3 contains two particular fatty acids that benefit the human body greatly. You should therefore take note that fatty fish and fish oils contain Eicosapentaenoic acid (EPA) and Docosahexaenoic acid (DHA). These are the fatty acids that have been observed to provide many benefits to the human body.

These fatty acids have been linked to helping prevent heart disease, cancer, and many other diseases. DHA is also required by the human brain. Therefore, the regular and repeated consumption of Omega 3 fish oils can greatly help enhance the quality of your life for the better.

The two essential fatty acids, EPA and DHA, are also helpful in preventing atherosclerosis, heart attacks, depression and various forms of cancer. Fish oil supplemented foods have also proven to be useful in treating illnesses like rheumatoid arthritis, diabetes, Reynaud's disease and ulcerative colitis. There are a lot more illnesses and situations in which intake of fish oil has proven to be significantly beneficial.

There are many reasons fish oil is good for your health. For one, the scientific world generally agrees that the Omega-3 fatty acids found in fish oil known as EPA and DHA promote a healthy vascular system. Also, the more fish oil absorbed by your body, the more "good" Eicosanoids your body will release. Eicosanoids are a type of hormone found in the body. There are both "good" and "bad" Eicosanoids. Fish oil helps to balance these levels, and in turn aids in such things as heart performance.

You can consume fish oil by eating the flesh of fatty fish or in the form of convenient fish oil supplements which may be in the form of liquids in a bottle or packaged in fish oil capsules

Getting Omega 3 from flax seeds

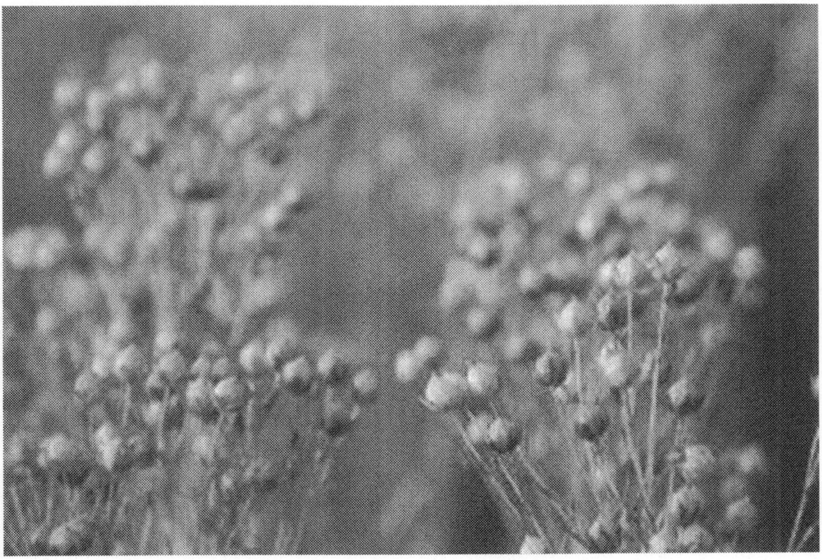

Flax seed has been a widely grown crop for thousands of years, and it is believed that it was one of the first plants that humans domesticated and farmed. It is one of the most versatile plants in the world, capable of being made into fabrics such as linen, medicines, high quality paper such as that used for money, soap, and all sorts of other things. The most useful thing that flax seed can be made into, however, is linseed oil, which is also known as flaxseed oil.

There are 2 types of Flaxseed. These are called 'Brown' and 'Golden' Flaxseed. Brown flax, can be eaten however, it is grown for the commercial Linseed Oil, paint, and solvents Industries. The Omega Golden Flax Seed was developed for human consumption and is preferred for the food market because of its nutty buttery flavor. The nutritional value of golden flaxseed and brown flaxseed are very similar if the samples are of the same quality. Quality is very important in determining the omega-3 and omega-6 content and overall nutritional value.

Linseed oil is one of the most commonly used vegetable oils. As well as being used in food, it has also been used as a finish and polish for wood and painted surfaces, in putty and caulk, and perhaps most notably in linoleum, which many people wrongly believe is made from man made materials. Linoleum is actually wood or cork dust on canvas, overlaid with solidified linseed oil, making an all natural floor covering that is especially suitable for people with allergies. Wood is also treated with linseed oil when making bats for some sports, including cricket.

The popularity of linseed oil for food preparation has been steadily growing again, as people have been paying more attention to the benefits of omega-3 fatty acids, which the oil is rich in, while also being low in the omega-6 fatty acids that many people are now trying to avoid. Some have come to use it as an alternative to cod liver oil, and it is readily edible poured straight onto salads. It has a nut like flavor. If you do not like the taste, though, capsules of the oil are also available. As most of the world's flax seed is cultivated in Europe, it is much cheaper there than elsewhere, but as a rule it should be cheaper than cod liver oil in almost all countries.

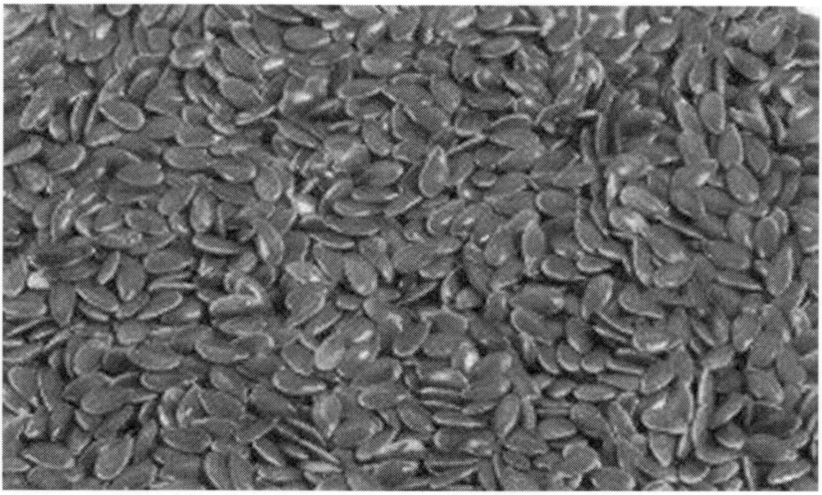

Flax seeds are a good source of Omega 3 fatty acids. In addition to this flax seeds are also rich in fiber, protein, vitamins and minerals. The fiber in the flax seeds can help stabilize blood sugar levels. The seeds are a great source for protein, for every 100 grams of the flax seeds you can get about 18 grams of protein. Flax seeds also contain vitamin E and B. The seeds are also rich in zinc, iron, copper, magnesium, nickel, calcium and many other essential minerals.

There are many benefits to adding flax seeds to your diet. Flax seeds can also help with your acne problems. The presence of fatty acids in the seeds helps to control the production of androgens, which causes acne.

There are also many ways of consuming the seeds. You can simply just chew them. You can grind the seeds to make a power. You can then mix the powder in juice, cereal or a non-dairy smoothie. If you want, you can also sprinkle the powder over a salad.

Golden flax can be purchased whole, ground and in oil form. It is recommended that you obtain golden flax seeds in the whole seed form as it provides the highest nutritional value. You should grind a portion of your golden flax seeds as needed. The golden flax seeds can be ground into a coarse powder form using a coffee grinder or electric flax grinder. Uncrushed flax seeds will not be digested and will thus pass through you undigested. This means that you will be missing out on any Omega 3 fatty acids that they contain.

There are many ways to consume golden flax seeds. Golden flax seeds add nutrition when added to bread dough, pancake, muffin or cookie mixes. When sprinkled on top of any of these before baking, they also add crunch and taste.

Whole golden flax seed, which is clean, dry and of good quality can be stored at room temperature for up to a year. For optimum freshness, ground flax seed should be ground as needed. This is important because they start to lose their healthy content as soon as they are ground. Unused ground flax seed can be refrigerated in an airtight container if it will be used in just a matter of days, or it can be stored in the freezer for about a month.

Ground flax can be added to your morning juice or chocolate milk by using a heaped tablespoon or two with your favorite beverage. You can also sprinkle ground flax on cereals or yogurt.

You should drink a lot of water after consuming flax seeds. You should also eat just the right amounts, which consists of no more then 3 tablespoons twice a day. If you exceed that by large amounts it can cause a toxic effect. As a result you should be careful.

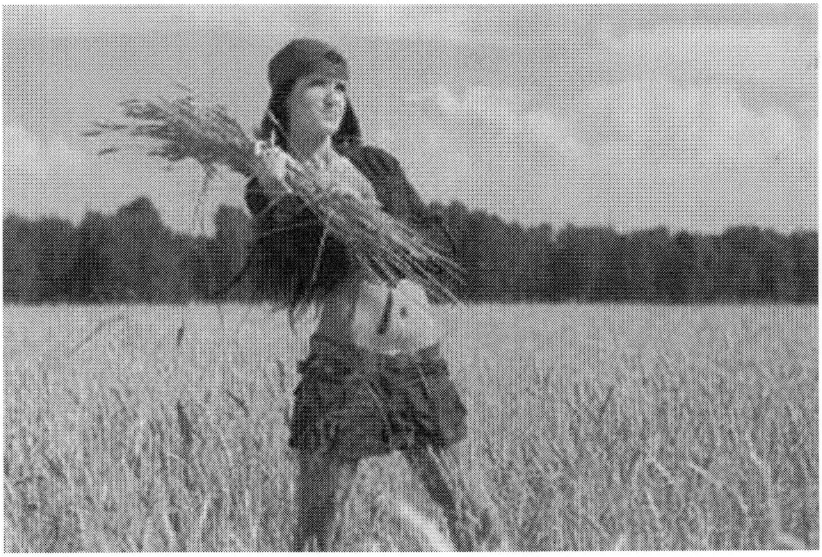

There are many great benefits for those who add flax seeds to their diets because they can help reduce your risk of cancer, heart disease, arthritis, and it can also be a natural laxative. Flax seed is essential for a well balanced and healthy body and good mental health. Everyone should add flax seed supplements to their own diet.

There are many different forms of flax seed to choose from including raw flax seeds, flax seed oil, and flax seed supplements. Raw flax seeds offer the best nutrients because they haven't lost anything while being processed. Many people increase their consumption of flax seed by grinding it and then sprinkling it on muesli, soup, salad, and even various casseroles. They can also add a nutty flavor to baked goods such as muffins or pancakes. Keep in mind that as soon as you cook flax seed some of the nutritional value is destroyed and there are less essential Omega 3 fatty acids.

Flax seed is a great alternative for other types of oils that you often use for muesli. There are great recipes to make a delicious spreads or mayonnaise from it as well. You can consume one tablespoon of it by itself each day if you prefer. Capsules and liquid supplements are a common daily routine for many who want to add more essential Omega 3 fatty acids to their diet.

Before you add flax seeds to your diet, you need to be aware of a couple of issues. If you consume too much flax seed you can gain weight, but that is true of most anything. Flax seeds can go bad quickly so don't buy too much at one time. Store them in a cool, dry, and dark location inside the refrigerator or freezer. After you have ground them you need to consume them within a few days. It is rare, but some people are allergic to flax seeds so if you have any type of reaction make sure you see a doctor immediately.

Essential Omega 3 fatty acids, Lignan, and Mucilage in flax seeds offer many great health benefits. Adding them to your diet in the form of seeds, oil, or supplements will help you feel your best physically and mentally. Be cautious if you have not taken them before as you could develop an allergic reaction. Always store them in a cool, dark, dry location and eat them as soon as you can.

Understanding why you eat certain foods is essential in maintaining life long health habits. Certainly, pleasing taste and visual appeal is one reason we make food choices. Eating flax seeds may not seem to be appealing; however, choosing foods that keep our body working as a finely tuned machine is also the goal that healthy minded individuals try to achieve.

Heart disease and omega fatty acids

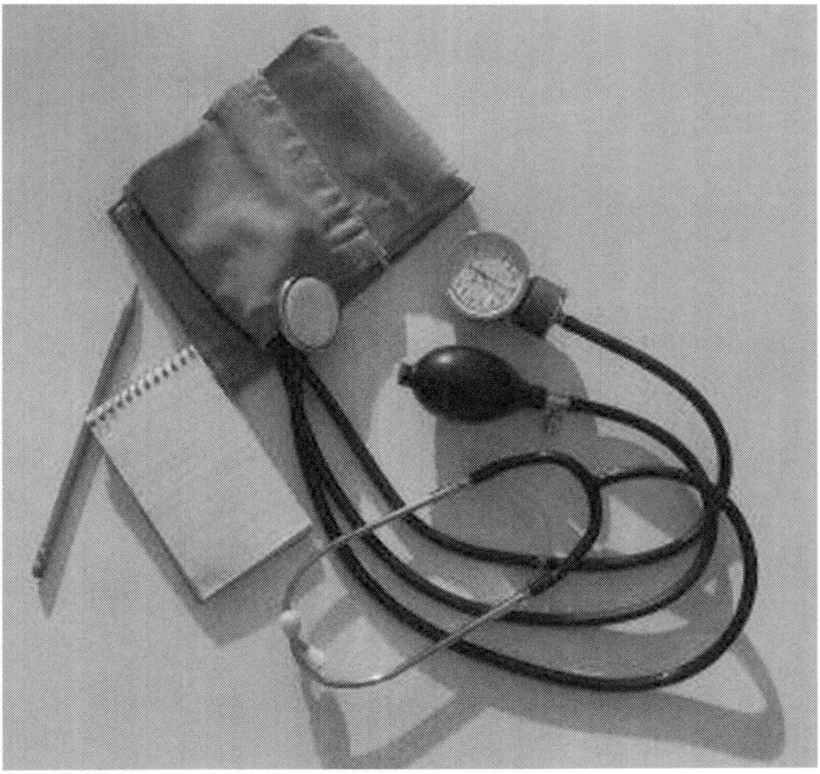

The benefits of fish oil are thought to be many, including a number of experts who believe that its consumption can help to regulate cholesterol. This problem affects many individuals and, if left untreated, can lead to more serious complications.

The heart is one of the most important parts of our body and having an unhealthy heart means having to suffer a rather limited life style and lifespan. Naturally, it's in our best interests to keep our heart happy and healthy and one way of doing that is eating food that contains fish oil.

According to the American Heart Association, daily consumption of the correct amount of fish oil can be beneficial for patients suffering from coronary heart disease. In addition, the United States National Institute of Health recommends fish oil for the prevention of cardiovascular disease and high blood pressure.

Studies have confirmed that for these reasons, fish oil can help to protect you from heart disease. A study done at Harvard University resulted in theconclusion that taking fish oil once a week lowered your chance of death from heart disease by 34 percent.

Physicians and scientists are of the same opinion, that one cause behind increasing cases of heart disease, hypertension or high blood pressure, obesity, diabetes, premature aging and certain kinds of cancer is none other than an imbalanced intake of omega-3 and omega-6 EFAs.

In the early 1970's a study on Greenland Eskimos revealed that one of the major reasons why they rarely suffer from heart diseases is because of their high fat diet which is mainly composed of fish.

The American Heart Association recommends the use of fish oils to help your heart's performance as long as you keep your dosage under 3 grams per day. They suggest an amount roughly between 0.5 to 1.8 grams per day. Clinical trials conducted so far have shown that Omega 3 fish oils can reduce cardiovascular problems including heart attacks, strokes, and even death.

The Japanese eat fish which contain high levels of omega 3 and this may explain why the Japanese population has very low levels of heart disease when compared to people in the USA. A study on Japanese omega 3 consumption was conducted by the University of Pittsburgh in 2008 and presented in the Journal of the American College of Cardiology. The death rated from coronary heart disease in Japan is less that half that found in America. The study compared blood levels of omega 3 with amounts of cholesterol buildup in arteries for Japanese, white American and Japanese American men. The men in the study were between the ages of 40 and 49. It was found that Japanese men had the smallest amount of cholesterol buildup in their arteries and twice as much omega 3 fatty acids in their blood serum compared to both the white Americans and the Japanese Americans. The results stayed the same even after adjustments to take into account other risk factors such as smoking, body mass index and diabetes.

The conclusion of the study was that high levels of omega 3 fatty acids have effects within the body that could help to stop the buildup of cholesterol in arteries. Although it is recommended that Americans should have fish at least two times a week this study suggests that increasing the amount still further would have a greater beneficial effect when it comes to heart disease.

It is interesting to note that the Japanese Americans had similar or even greater cholesterol build up in arteries when compared to white Americans. This suggests that the observed lower levels of cholesterol buildup in Japan are diet related rather than genetic in nature.

In the Greek city of Athens a study showed there was a direct relationship between high fish diet and reduced inflammation of blood vessels. The results revealed that those who ate more fish than the others had a lower level of C-reactive protein and interleukin-6. These are factors that are commonly used to measure the likelihood of blood vessel inflammation. These benefits remained even when the various risks associated with high fish diet were taken into account.

Research has also shown that fish oils can help decrease the risk of arrhythmias, decrease triglyceride levels, reduce the growth rate of atherosclerotic plaque, and even slightly lower blood pressure. With all of these factors to consider, there is little doubt that the regular and responsible use of Omega 3 fish oils from raw foods and supplements can be of great benefit to your health.

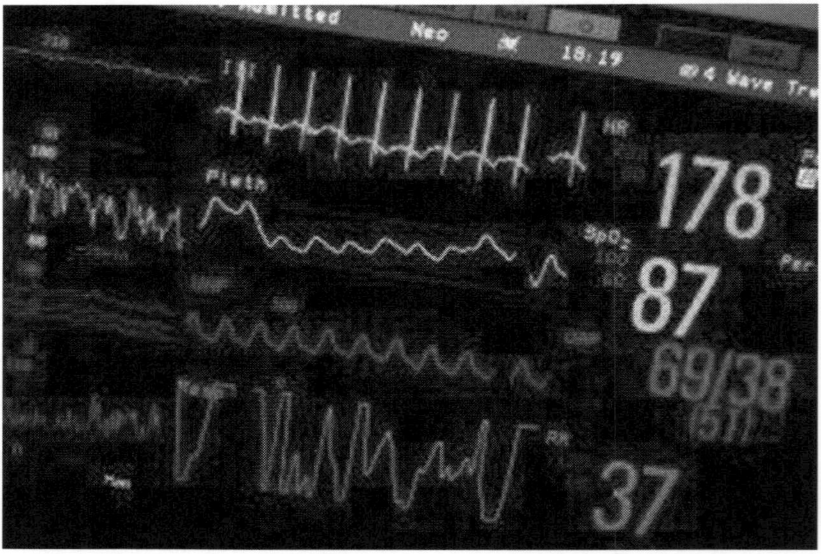

Some research on statin drugs show only a 1% reduction in arterial plaque. This could mean that instead of spending thousands of dollars on a prescription drug, you should at least consider a healthier and far less expensive dietary supplement like flax seed or fish oil.

The American Heart Association found that women with increased dietary intake of the isoflavones and lignans found in soy and flax seeds decreased their risk for atherosclerosis and arterial degeneration. Flax is by far the richest source of lignans, according to the Journal of the American College of Nutrition.

Like aspirin, omega-3s may reduce blood clotting and therefore reduce the chance of a fatal heart attack.

Flaxseeds and their oil may also lower total blood cholesterol, as well as just the bad LDL cholesterol. This should come as no big surprise, since any highly unsaturated oil will do that, particularly if substituted for saturated fats. The fiber in flaxseeds may also help against cholesterol. This is because the fiber traps the cholesterol stopping it from being taken into the body from the gut. This acts in the same way as oats do in preventing cholesterol absorption.

Studies at the University of Saskatchewan in 2009 concluded that flaxseed could improve the health of the heart and blood vessels. This is because the flax lignans contain secoisolariciresinol diglucoside which reduces the build up of atherosclerosis related to coronary heart disease. Studies have found that secoisolariciresinol diglucoside is a very strong compound when it comes to reducing high blood pressure. It also seems to protect the blood vessels around the heart from becoming blocked. This is the greatest cause of heart disease.

A study carried out by scientific teams in Sweden and the USA and published in 2009 in Medical News Today produced results that suggested that eating fatty fish and seafood containing omega 3 fatty acids could reduce the risks of suffering from heart failure. It was found that fatty fish and omega 3 containing fish oils could protect men from the risk of heart failure. This was the largest study of its kind. The results only related to men that consumed one serving of fatty fish each week and also consumed a moderate amount of omega 3 fatty acids from marine sources. This moderate amount is equivalent to about 0.3g of the oil each day.

Interestingly it was found that increasing the amount of these types of food that were consumed had no further beneficial effect. In fact the more that was eaten the more that the risk returned to the levels shown by low consumers of fatty fish and omega 3 fatty acids. In addition to this it was also discovered that taking supplements with omega 3 didn't produce the same results in men. The men in the study gained the majority of their omega 3 directly from fish and other marine foods.

Nearly 40 000 men between the ages of 45 and 79 were involved in the study. The researchers recorded details of the men's diet and then later tracked the end results by consulting patient registers giving causes of death. During the course of the study nearly 600 of the men without a previous heart condition went on to develop heart disease. Of these 34 actually died. The study therefore found that men who ate fatty fish once a week were twelve percent less likely to develop heart disease when compared to those men who never consumed fatty fish. When the results also took into consideration the consumption of marine omega3 fatty acids the results jumped to 33% less likely to develop heart disease.

It is not clear why increasing the amount of omega 3 had the negative results that were observed. As a result the recommendation from this report is to consume fatty fish and omega 3 in moderate amounts to get the best results in terms of heart conditions.

Preventing blood clots

Every minute of every day, our cells are busy breaking down the molecules of certain substances and building up the molecules of others. When we refuel our bodies with essential nutrients, the engine keeps working efficiently with minimal risk of breakdown. However, when we consistently try to refuel with foods of poor nutritional value the cells of your body start to work inefficiently and this may lead to various health problems.

Researchers at The University of Tromso in Norway have reported that the use of fish oil supplements lowers blood pressure significantly in people with high blood pressure.

Blood clots can form when the normal flow of blood is restricted by partial blockage of blood vessels with plaques of fatty material. These plaques are those associated with atherosclerosis. The plaques may contain a number of components including fats and platelets. The platelets can become sticky and this in turn tends to drag on the other blood cells as they pass over the blocked area. This is when the greatest risk of blood clots occurs.

As a result anything that can reduce the build up of these fatty plaques will lower the risk of blood clots, which could go on to cause strokes. Flax oil and fish oil can help to prevent the build up and blockage of vessels by the fatty plaques. Reducing blood pressure is an effective way to do this because then the blood isn't pressed up against the blood vessel walls with such force so fatty deposits aren't encouraged to build up.

Flaxseed for natural skin care

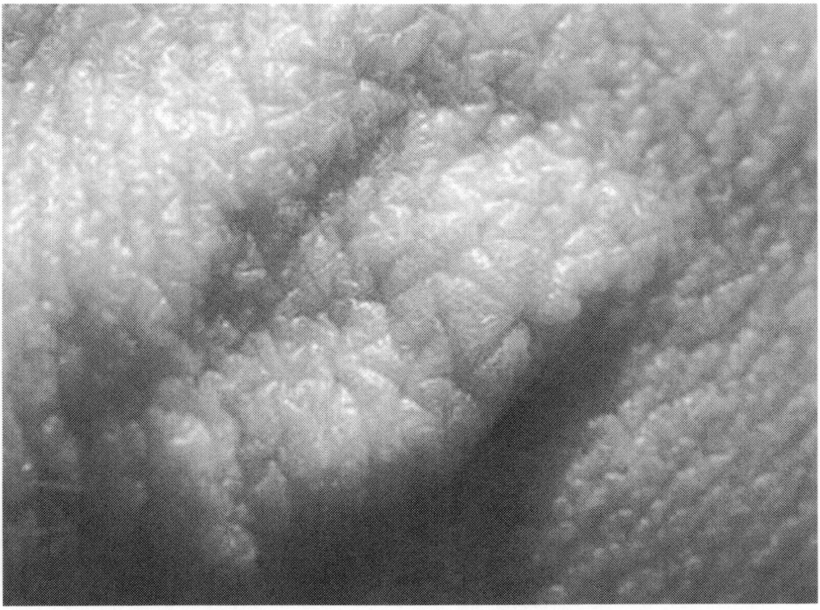

Flax seeds contain natural skin care components that are very rich in Omega-3 oils. These essential fatty acids are very important for our health and in particular for the skin. There are many skin problems such as acne, eczema, and psoriasis that may be caused by the lack of omega 3 essential fatty acids. As a rich source of omega 3 fatty acids, flax seed is able to replenish the correct body levels of these fats and so it can act as a natural skin care food.

A lot of people are also using flax seed oil directly on their skin in order to make it smoother and less dry. Some even report that directly applied flax seed reduces skin inflammations, but much more research is needed before we can know for sure whether this is true or brought on by a completely different factor, or simply a case of the placebo effect.

Skin products made from flax seed oil can easily become rancid, especially pure flax seed oil, where no preservatives have been added. Heat, light and oxygen will break down flax seed oil. To preserve its potency flax seed oil should be placed in an air-tight container that should be kept away from direct sunlight.

A spray top bottle with an extra lid is better than a normal bottle with a single lid because the spray construction reduces the possibility of air getting into the bottle. To prevent natural skin care products, such as flax seed oil, from turning bad you should always store them in the refrigerator. The best flax seed oil skin products are usually those processed at low temperatures in dark environments.

Flax oil and flax seeds are being rediscovered as true health foods. They definitely merit being included on any top ten list of natural skin care products that are good for everyone.

Flaxseed oil and acne

Symptoms of omega 3 fatty acid deficiency include dry skin, sticky platelets, and tissue inflammation. Given that inflammation is of particular concern for acne sufferers, it becomes easier to see why increasing the amount of omega 3 fatty acids in the diet remains a popular natural acne treatment.

Omega 3 fatty acids can be found in certain types of fish like salmon and mackerel, and flaxseed oil. And as well as reducing inflammation, omega 3's speed up healing, which is again important for acne sufferers. They also reduce platelet stickiness. Platelet stickiness becomes important beyond heart health when you consider that the blood cells carry the supply of oxygen to cells, including cells in our skin, and the cells that are involved in healing.

There are 3 types of omega 3 fatty acids that are significant for skin health. These are alpha linolenic acid (ALA or LNA), eicosapentaenoic acid (EPA), and docosahexanoic acid (DHA). ALA, or LNA, as it is often abbreviated to, is converted into EPA and DHA by the body. EPA and DHA are the forms in which the omega 3's are most easily used by the body. Supplementation with ALA has been found to reduce inflammation and improve dry skin.

Flaxseed oil is a very good source of ALA, containing an average of 55% and higher. But to carry out the conversions into EPA and DHA, the body needs to have good levels of zinc, magnesium, vitamin C, vitamin B3 and vitamin B6.

The recommended intake of ALA is about 2,220 mg per day. Higher doses are recommended to treat deficiencies, or some other conditions. There is no real standard recommendation for acne sufferers, simply because not enough studies have been done in relation to acne. However, doses of 3000 to 6000 mg per day are used to prevent and treat some chronic conditions.

Fish oil and weight loss

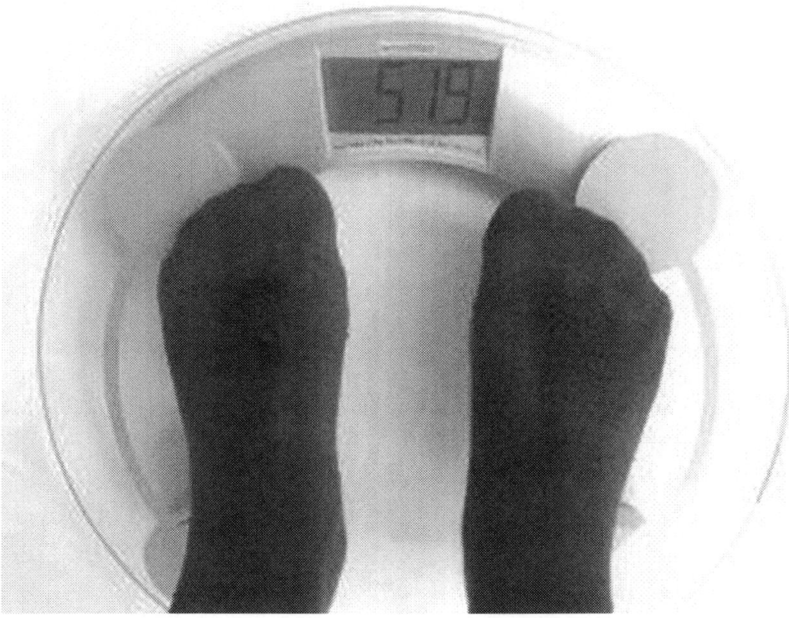

In Perth, Australia a study had revealed that fish consumption can be used against hypertension and obesity. Researchers of the UWA (University of Western Australia) have discovered that a weight loss diet which includes a regular amount of fish consumption can be quite effective in reducing blood pressure and improving glucose tolerance.

There are 3 main factors that are associated with the ability of people to lose weight. These are your metabolism, whether you are obese and being able to control your weight. Fish oil can help with all of these things.

Metabolism is something that most people have difficulty with. You can't see metabolism because it just describes the rate at which things happen inside your body. Some people have really slow metabolisms and they actually do have lots of difficulty getting rid of excess weight. For the majority of us, metabolism comes into play when we get those feelings of hunger after only just eating a big meal. It is hunger that makes us go and snack every now and then. We give into our metabolism all of the time.

This is where fish oil comes in. Omega 3 fatty acids can cause the 'I am full signal' which goes to the brain and causes it to stop sending the usual I am hungry reply that makes you eat more or go snacking.

Fish oils can therefore positively influence your metabolism and stop you from increasing in weight. An out of control metabolism can cause people to be overweight or even obese. It is also thought that Omega 3 oils can also cause the body to produce a hormone called Leptin which is involved in controlling metabolism as well.

Becoming obese is a difficult to understand process, and scientists think that there is a genetic link involved. After all, it can be observed that parents that are obese usually go on to produce children that have the same kinds of weight problems. However, even with this, people always wonder whether it is the genes or the learned bad eating habits that are responsible. In one animal experiment reproducing subjects were given food with reduced levels of omega 3 fats. It was found that obese individuals were formed within 3 generations. As a result Omega 3 could be the key to preventing obesity over the generations. It doesn't have to be passed on relentlessly to offspring.

The first stage in taking charge of your future is to focus on weight control. We all know that reducing calories and increasing levels of exercise are the backbone of any attempt to lose weight. In experiments, obese adults were given moderate amounts of exercise to do. There were two groups: one had omega 3 oils as part of their diet whereas the other group didn't. It was found that the group taking the Omega 3 lost a lot more weight than the group that didn't have it. As well as this, the weight loss was found to be focused more on the tummy region.

The conclusion to this is that it is thought that the Omega 3 helped special fat burning enzymes to be activated so that when combined with the exercise fat was more effectively used up. This in turn helped to increase the body's metabolic rate.

It has been found that fish oil can be seen to work better than just diet and exercise on its own. As a result if you are on a diet plan and you find that you are going no where with it or you have reached the calorie reduction plateau then why not try adding some fish oil to your diet. You might be surprised by what happens.

Asthma

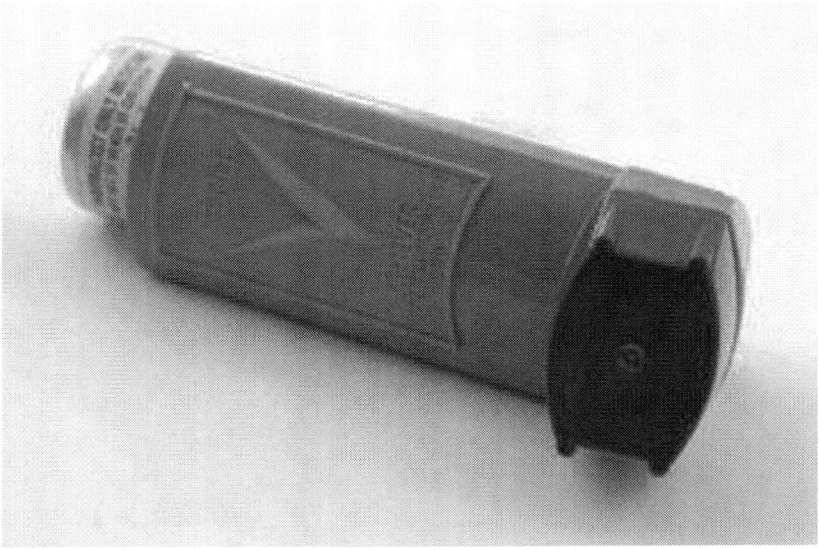

Asthma appears to be a modern disease with more and more children reporting problems with it. It seems to be closely related to allergy reactions which have also seen an increase in our modern world. A lot of people put this down to an increasing number of different natural and man made compounds that we are exposed to during our lifetime.

People suffering from respiratory problems like asthma tend to be perceived as unfit and unhealthy. Statistics show that approximately 20 to 25% of children today suffer one form of asthma or another at a certain point in their lives. As well as this, certain evidence also reveals a regular diet of food with high linoleic acid content as a possible reason behind it. This is an omega 6 related oil source. Consuming more omega 6 disturbs the natural balance with omega 3.

There has been a lot of research indicating that fish oil in the diet can reduce the occurrence of asthma especially in children. Researchers at the University of Wyoming conducted a study by giving a number of children a high fish diet while others continued with their regular diet. Results revealed that the participants who ate more fish were less prone to asthma attacks and were generally able to breathe more easily as well.

In Australia they have also seen an increase in asthma cases and it has now become a big health problem. At least 31% of children in Western Australia have been reported as having the condition. On top of this 12% of the population has some form of chronic inflammation of the airways. This includes reports of wheezing that is bad enough to prevent people getting enough sleep. Studies with Australian school children have shown that eating oily fish more than once a week can reduce the risk of asthma.

It has been suggested that the reason for the great increase in asthma rates in Australia is due to a change in the ratio of omega 6 fatty acids to omega 3 fatty acids in the diet. Whereas it used to 5 to 1 it is now 15 to 1 or higher. The studies that the Australian's undertook with the school children seem to bear out the reasoning behind this idea.

Another study in Japan backs up the findings of the Australian research. They found that giving fish oil supplements to children reduced the incidence of asthma symptoms with children who had already been hospitalized due to long term bronchial conditions.

Inflammation of the airways seems to be an important factor that one has to consider with asthma. As a result anything which acts as an anti inflammatory agent should help the condition. It just happens that the EPA and DHA components of fish oil are able to act in this way. They reduce the amount of cytokine produced by cells under stress. Cytokines are involved in the inflammation process.

Nervous system

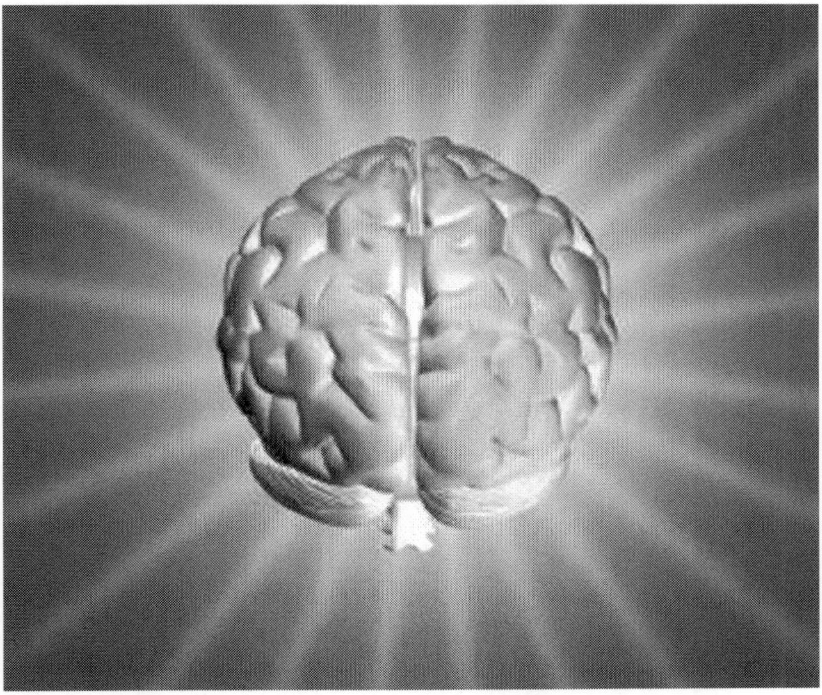

Doctors generally believe that the best way to treat mood, thought, and memory disorders is with pharmaceutical medicines that directly influence levels of brain chemicals such as serotonin, dopamine, and acetylcholine. Although these drugs have very important clinical uses, they are only part of the solution. A comprehensive approach to treating cognitive disorders should include foods and supplements that benefit the overall health of brain cells. These include omega-3 fatty acids found in flaxseed and fish.

One way to influence brain health through diet is to consume the right fats and oils. About 60 percent of the brain consists of lipids (fats) which make up the lining, or cell membrane, of every brain cell. The types of fats present in the brain influence its structure and function. How well your mind works depends, in the long run, on what you eat.

The brain controls and coordinates the body. It needs large quantities of oxygen supplied to it in order to perform all of its essential tasks. A network of blood vessels and fine capillaries are responsible for maintaining this good supply of oxygen. The brain uses at least 20% of the oxygen available to the whole of the body when it is at rest and not performing exercise. Healthy blood vessels are therefore very important for maintaining good functioning of the brain.

Fatty materials make up most of the brain structure. In particular, the transmission of messages along the nerves in the brain relies on a fatty insulating myelin sheath around the extended regions of the nerve cells. Essential fatty acids are needed to produce these parts of the brain and that fat has to come from the diet.

There have been studies performed involving people with conditions such as depression, attention deficit disorder and some dementia conditions. It has been found that there are links to these conditions and the lack of fatty acids. It has been found that boys with low levels of omega-3 fatty acids can have problems related to their behavior and learning. These boys are suffering from attention deficit hyperactivity disorder (ADHD).

There have also been studies into depression, where it has been found that there is a lot of evidence to support the idea that omega-3 essential fatty acids are important.

These fatty acids can be used to treat depression. Flaxseed is of course rich in this particular fatty acid.

It is believed that diets that have sufficient levels of the essential fatty acids omega 3 and omega 6 can help to keep the nerves in the brain working well. Without these the brain has to compensate by producing networks of brain cells that don't work as efficiently as normal. Over a long period of time the build up of these less efficient nerve pathways can lead to memory problems, mood swings and learning difficulties. This is because over time the brain has difficulty compensating for the inefficient systems.

Flaxseeds and fish oils are a good source of the omega 3 essential fatty acids and as a result it can be used to try and restore the balance within the body so that the brain has the correct building blocks to hopefully repair and damage that has been done.

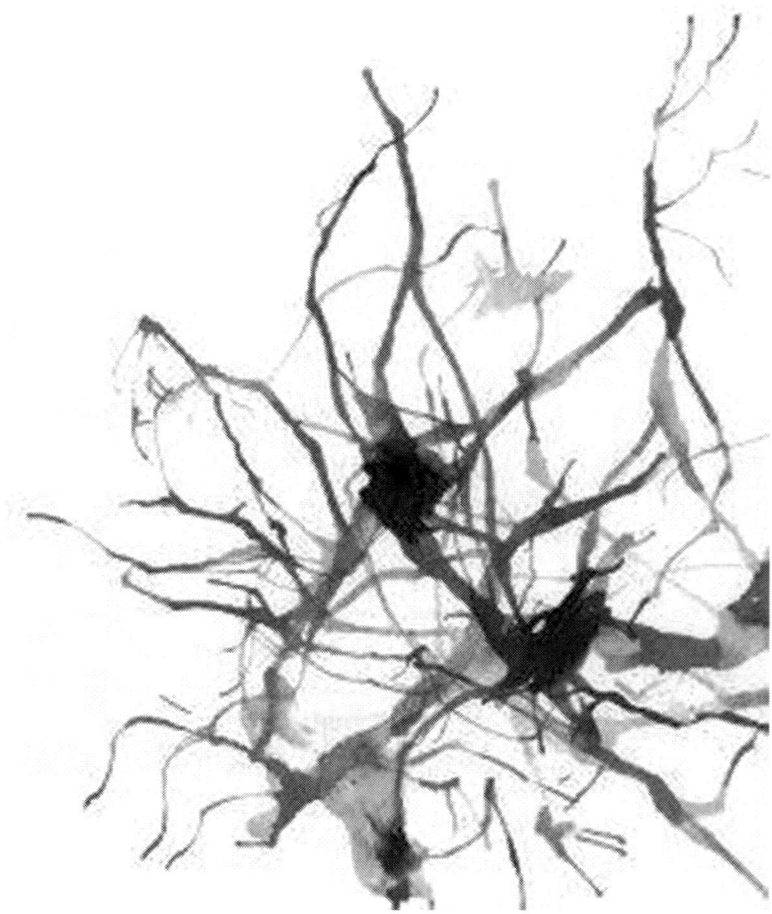

There are numerous benefits from fish oil that have been identified in scientific studies. There have even been studies that link low levels of omega 3 fatty acids with an increase in violent behavior among prisoners. Fish oil can help regulate the cholesterol in your body and this is thought to be one factor involved. There is also strong evidence to support the theory that the fatty acids found in fish oil are needed for the growth of neurons in the frontal cortex of the brain, which most neurologists believe is responsible for personal behavior and impulse control.

Fish oil has also been studied for its help with bipolar disorder. A Harvard study showed that the disorder could be treated with fish oil with remarkable success. The subjects found that their mood stabilized when taking fish oil. In addition to this the treatment didn't appear to have the side effects associated with other treatments such as Lithium. Lithium can lead to weight gain, tremors and cognitive dulling to mention just a few things. It also appears that the use of Omega 3 oils either on their own or with other treatments had positive effects with patients that were seemingly incurable. This enabled them to lead normal lives after their mood had been stabilized. It should be noted that the patients were given high doses of fish oils and this can only be safely done with high quality refined oils.

Low levels of DHA in the brain have been linked to depression, schizophrenia, memory loss, and an increased chance of being stricken with Alzheimer's disease. Experiments with rats have shown that when the animals were given fish oil supplements during the whole of their lives that it acted as an antidepressant. Chemicals associated with depression were measured in the rat brains after getting them to do activities such as mazes that could give rise to the condition. It was also discovered that the rats had elevated concentrations of EPA and DHA in the cerebral cortex and hippocampus parts of the brain. It was concluded that these were responsible for the antidepressant effects that were observed.

In September 2005, Louisiana State University conducted a study that resulted in findings to support a theory that fish oil may prevent the brain from developing cognitive problems that are associated with Alzheimer's disease. This illness, which is common among the elderly, causes an individual to gradually lose his or her memory.

In other studies people who had age determined memory problems and were over 55 years of age were given fish oil supplements. It was found that errors in learning and memory skills tests were reduced by 50%. The people were compared to another group that didn't take the supplement. The results were considered to be the same as people who were at least 3 years younger than the subjects involved. Unfortunately, a second study showed that the supplements didn't appear to slow down the onset of Alzheimer's disease where the subjects had moderate symptoms of the condition.

A recent study done by the University of Iowa has suggested that Omega 3 has little effect on the decline in memory ability in older women. The study involved over 2000 women aged between 65 and 80. The women had blood tests at the start of the study to determine their levels of Omega 3. Each year for 6 years the women were given thinking and memory skills tests to complete. These memory test results showed that there was no difference between the women with high levels of omega 3 in their blood and those that had low levels. In addition to this there were no differences in how the speed of thinking was lost between the women either. Despite these results the doctors involved stated that this wasn't the complete answer to the relationship between Omega 3 and brain health. They pointed to an earlier study in Medical News Today journal which suggested a strong link between the consumption of Omega 3 and the improvement of memory in young adults. This study involved young men and women between the ages of 18 and 25. These individuals increased their consumption of omega 3 supplements for a period of 6 months. They were then given tests to assess their working memory. After the 6 month period the memory test and blood results were examined and it was found that there was an improvement in working memory among the individuals given the extra omega 3 supplements. This series of studies shows that the way that omega 3 affects the working of the brain seems to change depending on the age of the individuals involved.

Other previous studies have shown that people who eat a lot of fatty fish were less likely to develop Alzheimer's. Most people, however, don't eat enough fatty fish to actually benefit from the improvement it can give. Based on these studies it seems that it is not clear how much help fish oil supplements can be in combating this disease. While the Alzheimer's association is not prepared to recommend fish oil directly it is still thought that there might be some benefit and, with fish oil supplements freely available, people should make up their own minds and act accordingly.

Oils to help eye disease

A study has found that omega-3 fatty acids can reduce the risk of macular degeneration, which is an eye disease that destroys vision by damaging nerve cells in the eye. The results of a Harvard study, published in August 2001 in the Archives of Ophthalmology, showed that people with a high intake of omega-6 vegetable oils were more likely to develop macular degeneration, while those with a combination of lower omega-6 intake and high omega-3 intake were less likely to have the disease

As flaxseed and fish oil is rich in omega 3 fatty acids it can be included in the diet in order to redress the balance and restore the conditions necessary for maintaining the sensory nerve cells in the retina. In this way it is hoped that macular degeneration can be prevented in those people who are at risk from the condition.

The immune system and oils

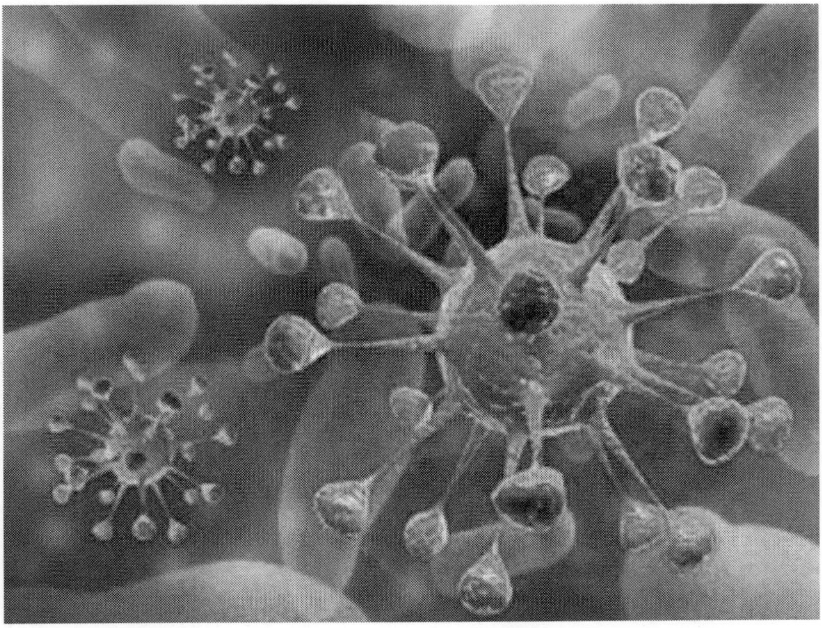

The immune system is important to protect the human body from the invasion of disease causing organisms such as bacteria and viruses. The lignans and alpha linolenic acid in flaxseed help to promote the healthy functioning of the immune system so that it can deal with these pathogenic organisms before they can establish in the body and cause disease.

The active ingredients in flax seeds also help to reduce inflammation and as a result it could be useful in the fight against autoimmune disorders such as lupus, psoriasis and rheumatoid arthritis. In these conditions the body appears to be attacked by its own immune system and inflammation results. Flax seed can help to reduce this inflammation.

Oils to help in the fight against cancer

There has been a great interest in the ability of fish oil to help in the prevention of cancer. There are many varied cancers with lots of different causes. Studies have been done on cancers to see what results the addition of fish oil to the diet can achieve.

Some cancers such as those of the esophagus or food pipe are very difficult to treat. There are certain conditions such as the refluxing of acid liquids from the stomach up through the esophagus towards the mouth that can lead to this particular cancer developing.

An enzyme called COX-2 has been identified as increasing in some pre cancer cells such as in the colon. It has also been found that fish oil can reduce the levels of this enzyme in the colon and in turn this has the effect of reducing the risk of colon cancer. COX-2 has also been identified in esophageal cells and as a result studies have been done into the effect of fish oil on this compound. The researchers found that people given regular small doses of fish oil went on to incorporate omega 3 fatty acids into their esophageal cells and this in turn lead to a reduction of the COX-2 enzyme. It is therefore suggested that fish oil supplements maybe a good thing to be taken to prevent this cancer especially for those who have the gastric refluxing condition.

More recently there has been interest in fish oils and breast cancer. Breast cancer is a very common cancer with over 200 000 new cases identified each year. Exposure to the hormone estrogen over long periods of time is thought to increase the risk of getting breast cancer. Women that are identified as being at risk from the disease are often prescribed the drug Tamoxifen. This drug works by inhibiting the action of estrogen in promoting this cancer. In experiments with rats it has been found that when tumors are being treated with Tamoxifen the addition of fish oil to the diet meant that the tumor became less aggressive and more responsive to the actions of Tamoxifen. In addition to this fish oil also appears to boost the actions of genes related to the immune response to tumors in general. It also reduced inflammation in cancer areas. Inflammation tends to reduce the ability of cells to fight cancer and can also cause the spread of cancer to other tissues. More research is now needed to see if the same ideas work in Women and whether Omega 3 oil can be used as a simple non toxic enhancer of Tamoxifen's ability to deal with breast cancer.

One of the keys to surviving cancer is the ability to maintain a healthy body weight. This is especially the case for the end stage of cancer patients. They get wasting syndrome where there is a loss of weight, mass of muscle and appetite. The loss of appetite just compounds matters as no new nutrients are taken in and muscle tissue is used up in essential respiration processes. Patients with a good body mass do better when treated and have a better chance of recovering from the cancer. They also have a better quality of life.

In studies with fish oil it was found that those who took a supplement for at least ten weeks maintained or even gained in the mass of their muscles. Those who took nothing usually lost muscle mass. It is thought that muscle mass tends to be lost due to inflammation which is a reaction of the body to the cancer. Fish oils disrupt the inflammation which in turn has a positive effect on body mass. The loss of muscle and fat reserves is bad for cancer patients because it gets in the way of their ability to cope with and respond to the actual cancer treatments. In a previous study involving pancreatic cancer patients it was found that fish oil could considerably improve patient appetite. This in turn means that more nutrients are entering the body.

Canadian research has found that fish oil supplements can increase the effectiveness of chemotherapy. The fish oil increased the destruction of cancer cells without affecting normal cells. The problem with chemotherapy is targeting it on the cancer cells rather than the normal cells of the body. The study was only done on patients with lung cancer that has resisted treatment and aimed more at palliative care. Survival rates are usually less than 30%. These were rates based on survival for 1 year. With the addition of fish oil survival rates for the year were increased to up to 60% and as a result fish oil can be seen as a way of extending the life of patients if they are being treated with chemotherapy.

On the negative side of things researchers in Seattle have discovered that fish oils are not so good for men with aggressive prostate cancer. Men with high DHA levels from fish oil were two and a half times greater at risk of developing the aggressive form of prostate cancer. These studies seem to contradict the usual feelings that fish oil is good at preventing cancer. Indeed in the normal forms of this disease fish oil was still found to be beneficial. It is only the aggressive form that seems to respond in this way.

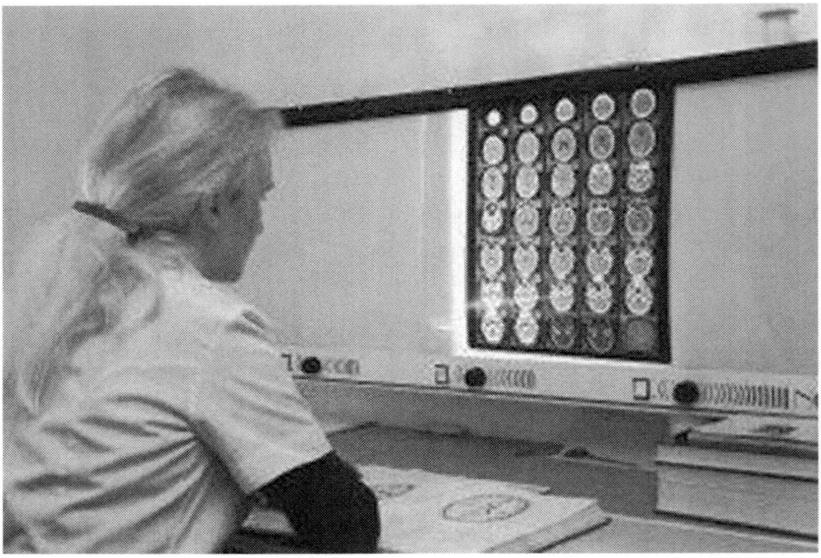

Recently small studies of cancer patients who consumed flaxseeds have produced some encouraging results:

In one study men with prostate cancer who ate an ounce of ground flaxseeds (almost three tablespoons) a day as part of a very low fat diet were able to slow the progress of their cancers between the time they were diagnosed and the time of surgery. A similar study of women awaiting surgery for breast cancer found that those who ate a flaxseed muffin daily (with about four tablespoons of ground flaxseeds per muffin) had a slower tumor growth rate. Studies of animals, too, suggest some anti cancer benefit from flaxseed. But it's always difficult to know whether it's the lignans that help, or some other element in the flaxseeds. And not all studies have yielded positive results.

Flaxseed pre lignans, converted in the intestines by bacteria into powerful anti cancer lignans, have been extremely efficient, in low doses, in killing the breast cancer cells in volunteer women. The results were nothing short of dramatic. The growth index in the cancer cells was reduced 34.2%, while the level of programmed cell death increased 30.7%. Women who expressed the HER2 metastatic oncogene saw its expression decrease by a dramatic 71%.

A lot of evidence relating to the anti cancer properties of flaxseed and flaxseed oil have been obtained from research on animals. Using mice and feeding them a diet with added flaxseed it has been found that there may be a reduction in the initiation, growth and spread of cancer related to the prostate gland. It also had the same kind of effect on breast and skin cancers.

Using rats scientists found that flaxseed managed to prevent polyp cancers developing in the intestine. It has also been discovered that flaxseed can slow the growth of breast cancer in mice. In the same study it managed to make the anti cancer drug tamoxifen more effective when applied to breast cells.

Laboratory cultivated cells have also been used in experiments. It has been found that flaxseed lignans can reduce the stickiness and movement of breast cancer cells. This means that it could help to reduce the ability of the cancer cells to infect other tissues.

There have been a few tests on humans and here are the results of these small trials. The first study involved giving 15 men a low fat diet with flaxseed added. The result of this was that the blood specific antigens to the prostate were reduced in level and the growth of pre cancer cells in the prostate was reduced. This means that it might be possible to reduce the risk of prostate cancer using flaxseed.

In the second trial using 25 men who already had prostate cancer a low fat diet with added ground flaxseed was used. In this case the growth rate of the cancer cells was reduced. There was also an increase in the death rate of cancer cells observed.

More research in humans is needed to determine the usefulness of flaxseed in cancer treatment and prevention. While animal and laboratory studies show promise, further studies are needed to determine whether the results apply to humans.

There are other studies that involve the assessment of diet in groups of people and the onset of colon cancer. The National Institute of Environmental Health Sciences performed such a study and presented their results in 2009. In this case they recruited approximately 2000 people to study. Half of these were cancer patients and the other half were healthy individuals that made up the control group. They were also made up of a mixture of black and white individuals.

They used a questionnaire based on specific foods and they collected information about the amounts and how often the individuals consumed these foods over a 12 month period. The individuals who consumed more omega 3 fatty acids in their food were found to have a lower risk of cancer of the large intestine. The people who consumed the most omega 3 had a 40 % lower risk of cancer. As a result it was suggested that consuming more foods with omega 3 such as from fish and sea food could help to prevent cancer of large intestine, otherwise known as bowel cancer. The results also showed that white people were more likely to get these benefits when compared to similar black individuals. There was no attempted explanation for this difference shown by the results of the study.

Pregnancy

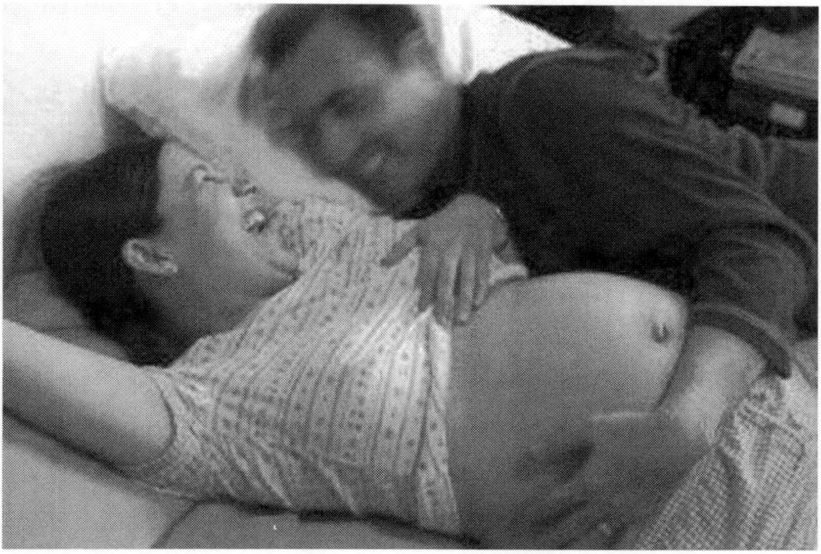

In the development of the fetus the circulation and nervous systems have to be constructed and this is where fish oil molecules become very important.

Omega 3 oils have been found to be important for the development of the nervous system and in turn the visual development of the baby. The normal western diet deficiency in these fish oils is compounded by the fact that levels of Omega 3 in pregnant women normally become reduced anyway, as the pregnancy progresses. This is bad news for the development of the fetus's nervous system.

Omega 3 is also used after the birth in the making of healthy breast milk and once again the baby's development depends on this. If mothers go on to have more pregnancies then they may end up with even further reduced levels of Omega 3 in their bodies. Adding fish oil supplements to the diet of pregnant women increases their levels of EPA and DHA. This in turn has a positive effect on the cognitive and visual development of the fetus and later the child.

There are also other positive contributions that fish oil can make. It has been found that omega 3 supplements may also reduce the instance of allergies and in children. During pregnancy fish oil supplements also seem to prevent the birth of premature babies as well as lowering the risk of preeclampsia. Babies also appear to have a higher birth weight. In terms of the mother, the addition of fish oil in the diet can also help to combat the usual depressions that occur after the birth. It is therefore important for mothers to continue taking the supplements after the birth, whether or not they are breast feeding. It is recommended that pregnant women have a consumption of 300 mg of DHA per day.

In terms of fresh fish pregnant women should avoid large predatory fish in case they have got a build up of mercury or other toxins in their bodies. Examples of these fish are shark, king mackerel and swordfish. The kinds of fish that are low in mercury include salmon, Pollock, catfish, tilapia and cod. It is generally recommended that it is safe to eat up to 12 ounces of fish per week.

In terms of fish oil supplements you should stick to those that are made from the body of the fish. These are the ones that are good for the development of the baby's brain and eyes and in the long term can help protect against heart disease and arthritis. You should avoid oil that has been made from the liver of the fish. Cod liver oil is an example of this and is high in the retinol form of vitamin A which could harm your baby.

Arthritis

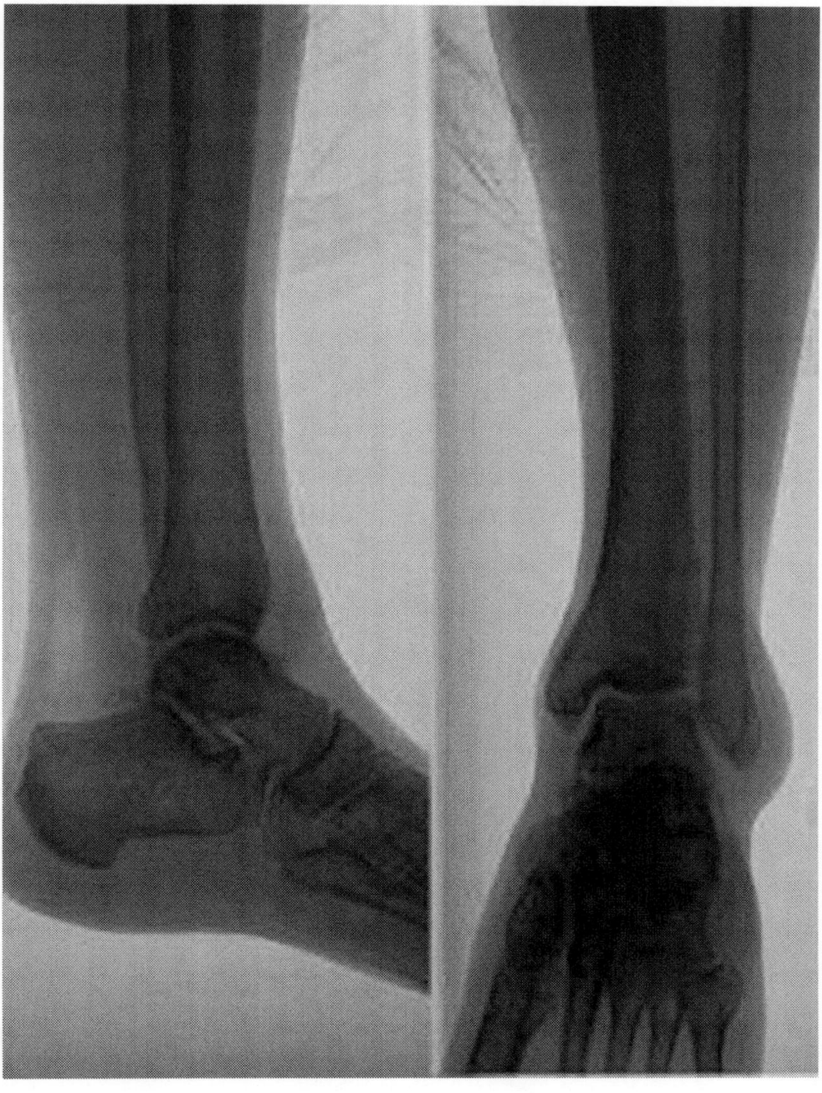

Arthritis isn't a disease that you can cure. It appears to be part of an autoimmune response where the body's own immune system attacks the joints. There are plenty of drugs that are available but all that you can hope for is a slowing down of the disease and some relief from the symptoms such as joint swelling and inflammation. One of the ways that the drugs work is to weaken the immune system so that it is less able to attack the joints while it is in its autoimmune phase. This however, then makes your body more vulnerable to attack from infection by bacteria and viruses. In addition to this, traditional arthritis drugs have many varying side effects including diarrhea, fever, stomach ulcers, headaches, rashes, kidney problems and bleeding gums. As well as this they can also increase the risks of getting certain cancers.

There has, of course, been a great interest in alternative treatments for arthritis so that the side effects of the drugs can be avoided. Taking Glucosamine tablets is one such suggestion but there is great doubt these days as to the effectiveness of this type of treatment. Despite this pharmacists are still making a lot of money selling these tablets.

Fish oil is another such alternative treatment. There have been a number of studies into the effectiveness of fish oils rich in omega 3 in their ability to deal with the symptoms of rheumatoid arthritis. Some of these studies show that the EPA and DHA in fish oil helps to a large degree in arthritis by reducing joint stiffness and joint aches and pains.

The University of Glasgow did a study into fish oil and found that supplements given to arthritis sufferers can result in a great reduction in morning stiffness and painful joints. The high concentrations of EPA and DHA in the fish oil block or suppress the over active inflammatory agents which cause rheumatoid arthritis.

Likewise a study with 50 patients in Australia found that fish oil supplements improved the condition of joints giving greater and less painful movements. This study compared those having the fish oil supplement with a control group taking a placebo. They found that it is necessary to make sure that omega 6 fatty acid intake is maintained at a low level so that the overall ratio of omega 6 to omega 3 was also kept at a low level. The omega 6 should be kept to less than 10g per day where as Omega 3 should be nearer 2.8g per day for person weighing 70 kg.

Although these and other studies have shown benefits to taking fish oil for arthritis it is a good idea to make sure that the higher quality oils from such fish as salmon and mackerel are used. There is still no clear advice as to whether fish oils can actually be used as an alternative to man made drugs in the treatment of arthritis. Even though the studies show some progress you have to remember that they will still have been taking the usual drugs as part of their treatment. Fish oils were given on top of these. Further studies are therefore needed to build on these results.

Oils and dogs

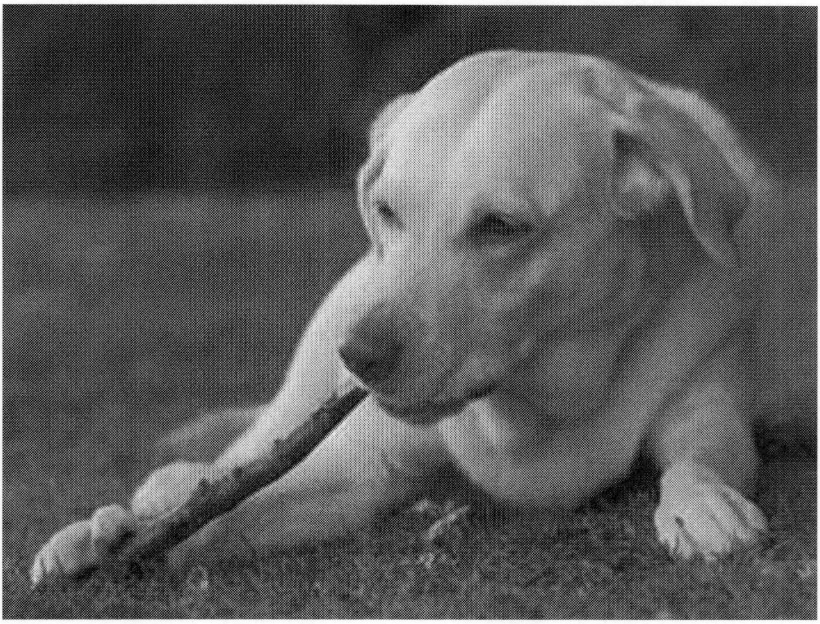

Omega 3 and Omega 6 fatty acids are just as important in the lives of our pets and in particular cats and dogs. They were first used to help treat allergies in pets but now are used to treat a whole range of animal problems. There are so many veterinarians now using fish oil to treat dermatological conditions in pets that it almost has to be considered as being conventional medicine albeit without drugs.

Processed food is the usual culprit in providing your pet with an inadequate diet. This is because they have a lot more omega 6 fatty acids when compared to the useful and good omega 3 fatty acids. This means that adding omega 3 fatty acid supplements to you pets diet is probably a good thing to do. The supplemented omega 3 leads to the production of eicosanoids which are responsible for reducing the itching and inflammation associated with dermatitis. Fatty acids are not the only cause of dermatitis and as a result they are often used together with other treatments to get an overall beneficial effect.

To aid the medication process the fish oils can be obtained in liquid form. This can be easier to administer to your pet compared to the usual capsule form. You can also get food which has the oils already added. These can be bought for example as medically produced dog foods that contain the fatty acids. These foods may in fact be prescribed by the veterinarian and obtained from them. This then becomes part of an anti inflammatory diet and is often prescribed for pets with allergies. There are of course additives and preservatives in these foods and you have to balance the merits of the fatty acids against these. You can, of course, produce a homemade natural diet for you pet and then add the fatty acid supplement yourself.

You should check the source of the fatty acids in any packaged processed food that you might be using. In some cases flaxseed oil is used and while it is a good source of Omega 3 and omega 6 fatty acids there can be some problems with different pets. This is because the alphalinoleic acid in flaxseed has to be converted by the animal into EPA and DHA. It is unfortunate that many animals including some dogs can't do this conversion. It is therefore far better to use fish oil as the supplement.

The actual effectiveness of any fish oil supplement depends on a number of issues which may work against them. One example of this is if the pet has any other disease as well as the normal allergy reaction. These diseases can also contribute to the itching that the pet is experiencing. These conditions include bacterial skin infections, yeast infections and flea infestations. It therefore stands to reason that these conditions need to be dealt with before you can expect the fish oil supplement to do its job.

While the use of fish oil supplements for pet skin conditions is widespread there is much controversy about its use with other pet problems. There is also debate about the correct amounts of these fatty acids that should be used. It has been suggested that as in humans there is an ideal ratio that should be used. Veterinarians and pet food producers have suggested that this should be five omega 6 to one omega 3. This appears to work for skin conditions but whether it is correct for all pets and all conditions is another story.

Veterinarians are now suggesting that fish oil can also be used for treating such pet conditions as arthritis, increased cholesterol and kidney disease. Undoubtedly some of these uses will become normal practice where as others will fall out of favor.

There are some basic benefits that dogs can get from fish oil supplements that increase the levels of omega 3 fatty acids in their diet. Studies in Italy with German shepherds have indicated that fish oil supplements can improve the behavior of dogs. This is really in terms of their temperament. They are less likely to show aggressive behavior. It is thought that this is because fatty acids are needed for the health of nerve cell membranes. If your dog is aggressive it could be due to a lack of omega 3 so it could be a good idea is to try some supplements of fish oil and see if the dog's behavior improves.

Not only can fish oil help with skin allergies it can also improve the look of the dog's coat and reduce hair loss. Nails are related to hair in their chemical make up and likewise fish oils can help improve nail health by strengthening them. It therefore helps to prevent cracked and split nails.

Just as described in the case of humans, fish oils can help with heart health in dogs. It can help improve cholesterol levels and prevent heart attacks and strokes. Likewise, fish oil helps with joint health in dogs as it does in humans.

Fish oil and cats

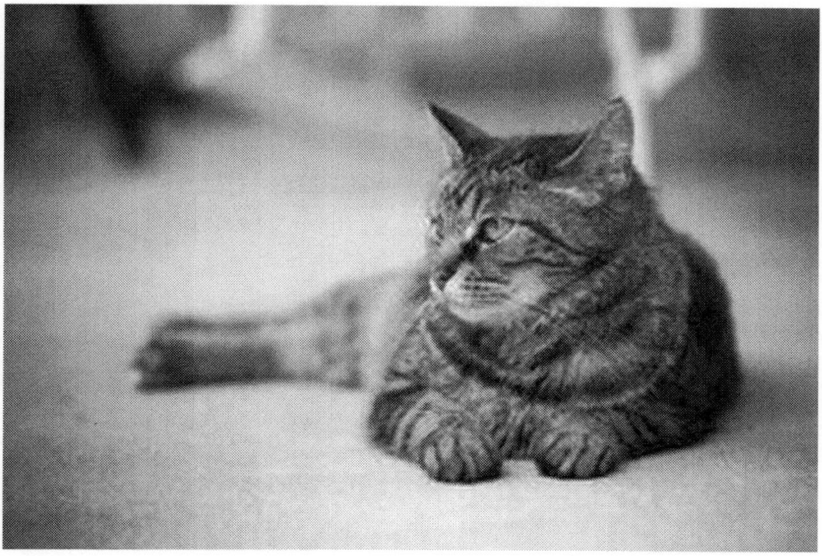

In cats a daily supplement of fish oil can have a significant affect on quality of life. The extent of the health benefits for cats from fish oil can be quite huge and includes prevention of heart disease, better vision and thinking ability. Also of importance is the treatment of arthritis and joint problems in general. The immune system is improved and cancer can be prevented

For older cats a daily fish oil supplement can help those that are suffering from arthritis. It can help restore joint movement and the cat will appear to be much younger in just a few weeks. Fish oil is also very good for helping with the cat's skin. It can help heal dry irritated areas especially where hair has been lost. It will help prevent them from having to scratch the area and thereby promote healthy skin growth and a healthy coat. In addition to this studies have shown that fish oil can stop eye disease and help prevent cancers forming and growing.

Don't be fooled by thinking that you need special oils for cats. In general the same ones that are used for humans can be used and these tend to be cheaper. You also don't need to give as much supplement as humans due to the lower body mass of the cat.

You should look for oils with high DHA levels because DHA is the most important component for the health of your cat. If you are using capsules then ones that have 250mg of DHA are the most appropriate. Giving fish oil will mean that your cat will live longer and have a healthier life by avoiding a lot of those degenerative diseases that harm cats.

Fish oils or Flaxseed?

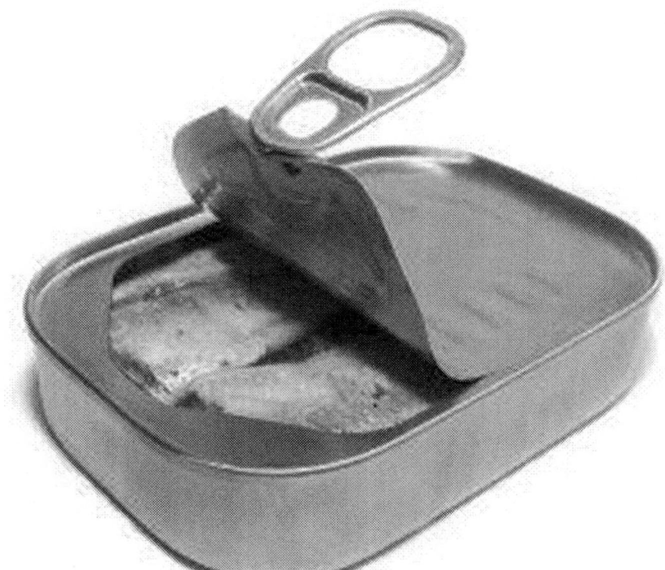

Fish oil versus Flaxseed oil

What is the opinion on fish oil supplements, and why not just take flaxseed oil since it has omega 3s? How much is needed to take daily?

The answer is really very simple. There are several Omega 3 fatty acids. They are named ALA (alpha linolenic acid), EPA (eicosapentanoic acid) and DHA (docosahexanoic acid). ALA is found in flaxseed oil whereas EPA and DHA are found in fish oils. ALA is able to convert into EPA and then into DHA, but this takes several enzymatic steps in the body and not everyone efficiently converts ALA into EPA and DHA, particularly with aging.

Lignans are a type of fiber, and at the same time a type of phytoestrogen which is a chemical similar to the human hormone estrogen. Flaxseeds are the richest source of lignans. When you eat lignans, bacteria in the digestive tract convert them into estrogen-like substances called enterodiol and enterolactone, which are thought to have anti tumor effects. Lignans and other flaxseed components may also have antioxidant properties, that is, they may reduce the activity of cell damaging free radicals.

Flaxseeds have a pleasant, nutty flavor and taste good sprinkled on salads, cooked vegetables, or cereals. The oil is quite tasty, too, though sometimes more expensive than other cheaper oils.

In addition to the omega-3s, the remaining two components of flaxseed, which are lignans and fiber are being studied for their health benefits as well according to the Flax Council of Canada. Lignans, for example, act as both phytoestrogens and antioxidants, while the fiber contained in the flaxseed is of both the soluble and insoluble type. Flax is an interesting mixture of nutrients and other components.

For vegetarians, obviously, flaxseed is a good choice but it isn't the only one as dark green leafed vegetables such as spinach and basil are also good sources of omega 3. Plant sources of omega 3 also don't have the mercury pollutant problems that have to be considered when choosing some fish sources for the oil.

Supplements

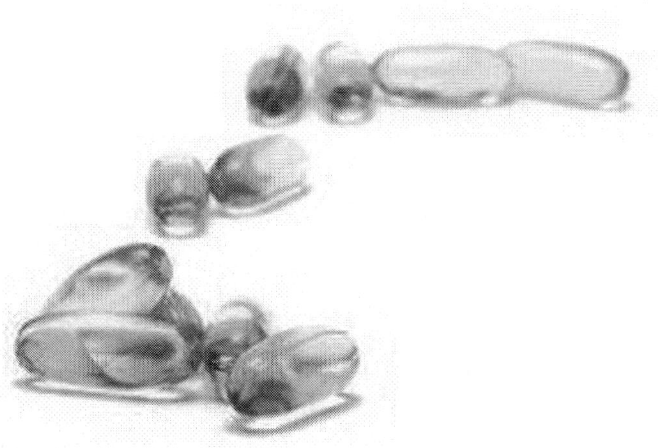

When buying fish oil supplements, make sure that the label states that the product is distilled, free of mercury and any other toxins, and that the product is USP certified.

The purity of the fish oil you are taking is a key factor in its benefits for your health. To make pharmaceutical-grade fish oil, you're required to put the raw product through substantial purification processes. 100 gallons of health-food grade fish oil results in merely one gallon of pharmaceutical grade fish oil. This pharmaceutical grade oil possesses about twice the EPA and DHA as the standard health food grade fish oil.

Apart from consuming fish on a daily basis, fish oil is available as dietary supplements and may be purchased at many locations. In certain cases, fish oil may require a doctor's prescription if the product is of pharmaceutical quality. It is important that individuals read the label and instructions carefully before using any medication or dietary supplement, including fish oil. It is also equally important that individuals inform their doctor of any current health problems or medications that they are currently taking.

When buying fish oil you can perform some simple checks to see if it is of the highest quality. The first thing to do is to check that the manufacturing process states that the oil is free of toxins. You can then smell the oil. If the oil smells fishy it is an indication that it has started to degrade and become rancid. High quality fresh oil should not smell fishy at all. You can then taste the oil. Once again the highest quality oils should not taste fishy. You should avoid oils that have strong flavors added to them as this is probably trying to hide the fact that the oils have actually gone rancid.

Side effects

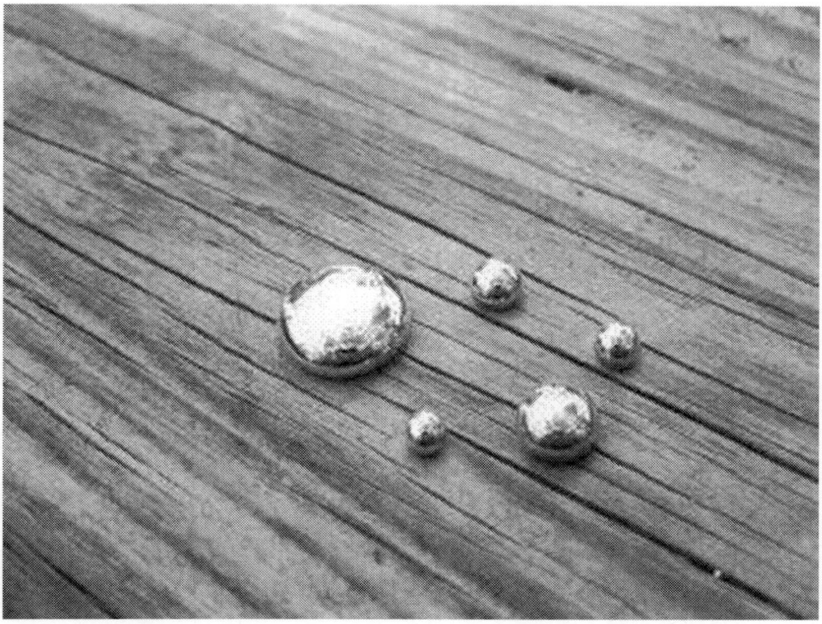

The American Heart Association says that high levels of omega-3 fatty acid intake may increase the risk of dangerous side effects, including a stroke. The liver of fish can contain dangerous levels of Vitamin A and this should be taken into consideration when selecting oil as a supplement.

As the name implies, fish oil is oil that is removed from the tissues of oily fish and is often recommended as part of a healthy diet program. Many nutritionists recommend that individuals eat fish at least once a week, but emphasis must be placed on the importance of avoiding fish that contain certain harmful contaminants. In avoiding predatory fish, such as sharks and others, individuals will prevent the consumption of unhealthy substances which can accumulate due to the fish's predatory lifestyle.

Some people say that there is a problem with eating fresh fish and mercury contamination. The mercury levels that are prevalent in almost all fresh fish these days can be very detrimental to your health. These fish are usually predators, and as such they may accumulate toxins and harmful chemicals by eating other fish which have these toxins in their body. The FDA has a recommendation concerning the consumption of these fish, because many of these fish have things like mercury, dioxin, Chlordane, and PCBs, built up in their fatty tissues. Because of these issues, many people are turning to fish oil supplements to get the benefits of fish oil without the contamination risks. To this end companies have manufactured fish oils that are mercury free by processing the oils that naturally occur in the fish

While flax seed is believed to be safe in general, there are potential risks that consumers should consider. As is the case with many ingredients and treatment products, there have been serious allergic reactions that have been reported by flax seed users. In addition, individuals who are already taking any type of medication must consult a physician before using flax seed or flax seed oil, which may interfere with the effects of other medicine. There are certain individuals who should consider avoiding flax seed and flax seed oil altogether, including women who are pregnant or breast-feeding. In addition, flax seed may be dangerous for anyone with a history of certain types of cancer or diabetes and other specific ailments.

Recent research has identified an indication that taking too much omega 3 in the form of supplements could be a problem for some men. It has been found that men with high levels of omega 3 in their blood could be at a 43% higher risk of developing prostate cancer. This is an indication that the over use of supplements isn't a good idea. If men stick to the recommended doses of these supplements there shouldn't be a problem.

The extra amount of omega 3 in these men was equivalent to eating over 2 additional potions of salmon each week. This research was undertaken at the Fred Hutchinson Cancer Research Center which is located in Seattle. They compared the levels of Omega 3 in the blood from cancer patients with a healthy control group of the population. These results back up a previous study that the same research center did in 2011. Despite this, the results of other studies across the world haven't been in agreement with these findings and as a result the evidence for a link with prostate cancer is still confusing. It isn't clear how excess omega 3 might promote this type of cancer but it is thought that it leads to the body converting fatty acids into compounds that are able to damage cells and DNA as well as suppressing the immune system.

The advice from this study is that Omega 3 still has many health benefits and should be included in a balanced diet. People should, however, avoid the over use of Omega 3 supplements. It should be noted that although this study appears to have produced some useful information there has been a lot of criticism of its validity from doctors and scientists alike.

Example recipes

Salmon with a ginger and garlic sauce

Ingredients

2 salmon fillets
3 oz butter
1 tbsp soy sauce
1 clove garlic
1 inch fresh ginger
1 1/2 tsp brown sugar
1 tbsp lemon juice

Method

Grate the garlic and chop the ginger.

Put the salmon fillets on a grill pan and place under a preheated hot grill. Cook the salmon for about 5 minutes on each side or until they are done to your personal taste.

While the salmon is cooking place the butter, soy sauce, grated garlic, ginger, brown sugar and lemon juice into a small saucepan. Heat the mixture on a low heat while stirring. Once the butter is melted and all the ingredients are well combined pour the mixture over the cooked salmon fillets and serve while still hot.

Stuffed and grilled sardines

Ingredients

6 tbsp of mixed chopped fresh parsley, chives and basil
1 tbsp Dijon mustard
1/2 lemon
12 fresh sardines
Salt and black pepper
Extra virgin olive oil for brushing
Lemon wedges

Method

Juice the half lemon.

Mix the lemon juice, herbs and mustard in a small bowl.

Gut and clean the sardines. Rinse them and then pat them dry with paper towels. Scatter salt and pepper into the cavities where the guts were removed. Put equal amounts of the herb mixture into the gut cavities using a spoon.

Brush the sardines with olive oil and then place the sardines on a hot preheated grill and cook until each side is browned. Make sure that the fish is cooked through before removing the fish from the grill and serving on plates with a sprinkle of salt and pepper and a squeeze of lemon. Try serving with crusty whole meal rustic bread.

Fried herby smelt

Ingredients

Frying oil
1 cup all purpose flour
2 tsp garlic powder
1 tsp salt
1 pound smelt
2 tbsp butter
1 handful fresh herbs
1 clove garlic
1 whole chili
Salt and pepper
1 lemon

Method

Mince or finely chop the fresh herbs and the chili pepper.

Mix the flour, garlic powder and salt together and place the mixture into a wide shallow bowl.

Halve the lemon and then squeeze the one half of the lemon and retain the juice for later. Cut the other half of lemon into wedges for the garnish.

Add enough of the frying oil to reach a half inch up the sides of a deep frying pan. Heat the frying oil until it is hot enough to bubble and lightly brown the flour when small bits are dropped into it.

Dip a smelt into the flour mixture and dredge it through the flour until it is coated on both sides. Carefully place the coated smelt into the hot oil. Continue to add more coated smelt to the oil making sure that they don't touch each other. Cook the smelt on each side for about two minutes. Place the cooked smelt on a wire rack to drain off the excess oil. Continue the process until all of the smelt are cooked.

Put the butter into a small frying pan on a medium heat. Once the butter has melted add the garlic and chili. Once the garlic aroma becomes apparent add salt and pepper seasoning and the juice from the half lemon. Next turn off the heat and stir in the chopped fresh herbs. Put the cooked and drained smelt onto plates and then pour the hot butter herb sauce over them. Serve the plates straight away with lemon wedges.

Turkish fried anchovy

Ingredients

1 pound fresh or frozen anchovies
1/3 cup all purpose flour
1 tsp salt
1/2 cup sunflower oil
1 lemon
1 onion

Method

Defrost the anchovies if you have the frozen ones.

Cut off the heads and then gut the anchovies. Wash them in cold water and leave them to drain. Next put them into a suitable sized bowl and sprinkle them with salt. Mix them together so that the salt combines with the anchovies.

Pour the oil into a large frying pan and place the pan on a medium heat. Put the flour onto a plate and the use the tail of each fish to dredge it through the flour. Shake off the excess flour and then place each into the hot oil. Cook the anchovies for about 5 minutes or until they go a fried red color. Half way through cooking the fish turn them over so that both sides get cooked. Once they are cooked place them on paper towels to help get rid of the excess oil. Serve the cooked anchovies with lemon slices and roughly chopped onion.

Baked mackerel

Ingredients

2 ripe tomatoes
1 red onion
200g small new potatoes
2 cloves garlic
1 small bay leaf
Handful fresh parsley
2 whole mackerel
1 tsp English mustard
5 tbsp extra virgin olive oil
1 lemon
Salt and pepper seasoning

Method

Halve the tomatoes.

Thinly slice the red onion and new potatoes.

Crush the garlic cloves.

Chop most of the parsley saving some for the garnish.

Remove the scales from the mackerel and then gut them.

Mix the mustard with 1 tbsp of the olive oil.

Cut the lemon into wedges.

Put the tomatoes, potatoes, onion, garlic, parsley and bay leaves into a large bowl together with 2 tbsp of the olive oil. Season to taste and mix together gently.

Put 3 cuts into each side of the mackerel using a sharp knife. Season the fish and then brush them with the olive oil and mustard mixture. Stuff the gut cavity of each fish with a mixture made up of chopped parsley and the majority of the lemon wedges. Save some of the lemon for the garnish.

Place the potato and tomato mixture on a baking dish and spread it out. Place the mackerel on the top of this and drizzle over the remaining 2 tbsp of olive oil. Put the baking dish into a preheated oven set to 220C and cook for about 20 minutes.

Serve with a garnish of parsley and the remaining lemon wedges.

Herrings with basil

Ingredients

4 herring fillets
4 tbsp extra virgin olive oil
2 tbsp wholegrain mustard
1 large bunch basil
1 tsp clear honey
1 lemon
Ground sea salt
Freshly ground black pepper

Method

Roughly tear the basil.

Grate the zest and squeeze the juice from the lemon.

Wash the fish with cold running water and make sure that any loose scales are removed.

Brush the fish with some of the olive oil and season with salt and pepper to taste

Make a dressing for the fish by whisking together the basil, mustard, lemon zest, lemon juice and the olive oil in a bowl. Season the dressing to taste with salt and pepper.

Place the fish fillets under a preheated grill set to high and cook for about 8 minutes or until the skin is browned and the flesh is white and firm. Just before serving the cooked fish spoon on the dressing.

Flax seed smoothie

Ingredients

2 tbsp flax seeds
1 cup vanilla flavored soya milk
1 tsp lemon juice
1 cup strawberries
1 banana
6 tsp sugar

Method

Roughly chop the strawberries and the banana.

Place the soya milk, lemon juice, flax seeds, banana and sugar into a blender and whizz it all up until it is smooth and frothy.

Pour the smoothie into 2 glasses and serve.

Flax seed Granola

Ingredients

2 tsp ground cinnamon
1/2 tsp ground ginger
1/4 tsp salt
3 tbsp honey
2 tbsp extra virgin olive oil
2 tbsp maple syrup
2 tbsp water
1 tsp vanilla
2 cups whole oats
1/2 cup chopped pecans
1/2 cup crisped rice cereal
1/4 cup milled flax seed

Method

Put the cinnamon, ginger, salt, honey, olive oil, maple syrup, vanilla and water into a large bowl and whisk them together. Add the oats, rice cereal, pecans and milled flax seeds and gently stir so combine.

Spread out the mixture on a parchment lined baking sheet. Put the baking sheet into a preheated oven set to 150C and bake until the granola is crisp and dry but not browned. This should take around 30 minutes. Allow the granola to cool before serving.

Flax seed muffins

Ingredients

1 1/2 cups whole wheat flour
1 1/2 cups milled flax seed
3/4 cup brown sugar
1 tbsp baking powder
3/4 tsp ground nutmeg
1 1/2 tsp ground cinnamon
2 cups milk
1 egg

Method

Mix the flour, flax seed, brown sugar, baking powder, nutmeg and cinnamon in a large bowl.

In a separate smaller bowl beat the egg and then add the milk and stir to combine.

Add the wet ingredients to the dry ingredients in the large bowl. Stir until the dry ingredients are moistened.

Use non stick muffin pans and fill the tins so that they are three quarters filled. Place the muffin tins in to preheated oven set to 180C. Cook the muffins for about 30 minutes or until they are light brown on the top. Once they are cooked place the muffins on cooling racks. Serve when cool.

Conclusion

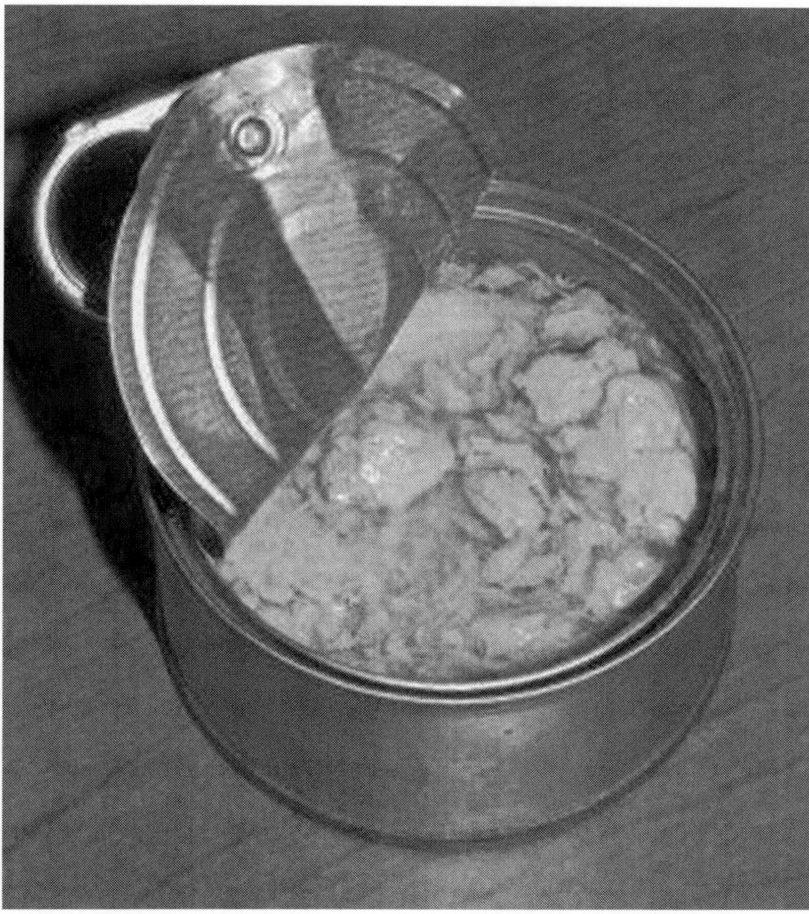

There is a lot of evidence that fish oil can promote health in both humans and pets such as dogs and cats. The basic active component of fish oil is omega 3 fatty acid and it is this that is lacking in modern diets whether they are for humans or pets. One of the main reasons for this is the facts that a lot of vegetable oils are used, which have a higher proportion of omega 6 fatty acids. It is the balance of omega 6 oils to omega 3 that is important. With an increase in omega 6 intake it means that extra omega 3 oil is needed to redress the balance.

You can simply take fish oil supplements or change your diet to include more fatty fish. If you go the natural fish way then you have to be careful when eating carnivorous fish as they may have accumulated mercury and other toxins in their flesh. Although fish oils show all of these health benefits they often work together with other substances and treatments in the body. They often work by enhancing processes that are already taking place in the body. Fish oil isn't often given as a prescribed medicine so it is up to the individual to buy supplements or change their diet in order to get more of the good omega 3 fatty acids.

It appears that getting omega 3 from a raw food source may be better than using refined supplements. This is probably due to the fact that the food contains other active ingredients that work together with the omega 3 oils in the food.

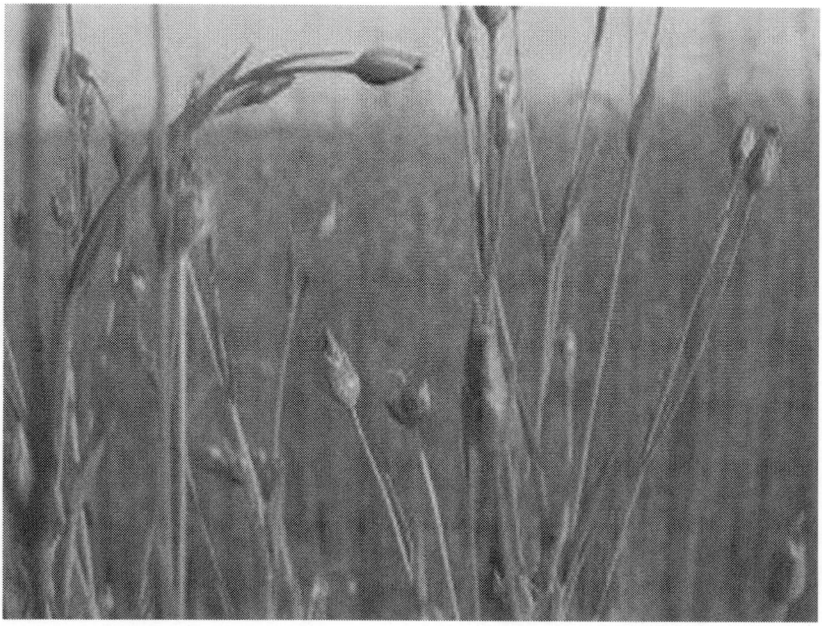

Flax seed oil has a history that is rich with it used as health treatments and it is believed to help in the prevention of certain illnesses. Flax seed oil is sold as a liquid, but must remain refrigerated at all times. Recent research studies have indicated that flaxseed oil may help to reduce high blood pressure, lessen high cholesterol and is currently being evaluated for its potential to prevent cancer.

The key to flax seed oil and its healthy benefits is that it contains essential fatty acids, which are especially valuable since the body needs them in order to function properly. The body, however, is unable to manufacture essential fatty acids on it's own and receives benefits from products containing such ingredients. One such benefit is derived from one of the essential fatty acids found in flax seed oil, which is believed to reduce the risk of heart disease and various other ailments.

Flax seed oil also provides a rich source of lignans, which are believed to possibly prevent certain types of cancer and help to fight against certain infections, including both bacterial and viral ones. Among its specific benefits, flax seed oil is thought to aid in the reduction of high cholesterol, control high blood pressure and protect against heart disease. Some studies have shown that lowering cholesterol may also reduce the risk of heart disease.

Flax seed oil is believed to help in reducing the inflammation resulting from gout, which often presents itself with sudden and severe joint pain or swelling. By reducing the discomfort of these symptoms, the individual may find relief from the sudden onset of gout. Because flax seed oil is a fiber product, it is often associated with relieving constipation and may even ease an upset stomach.

Together with its many believed benefits on the inside of the body, flax seed oil is thought to promote many cosmetic improvements on the outside as well. In addition to the treatment of acne, eczema and sunburns, flax seed oil is also believed to promote healthy hair and nails. The lignans found in flax seed oil are also thought to protect against many aging effects and a variety of other ailments. Flax seed oil is also believed to help soften dry skin when applied externally to the affected area, but may also prove beneficial for aching or injured skin.

About the Author

Ellen Vincent has written 2 other books. The first book complements this 'Green Smoothie Recipes' book because it gives more of the background as to why green smoothies are so healthy and how to make them. The second book details the health benefits of Apple cider vinegar. Both books are published as paperbacks and on the kindle platform.

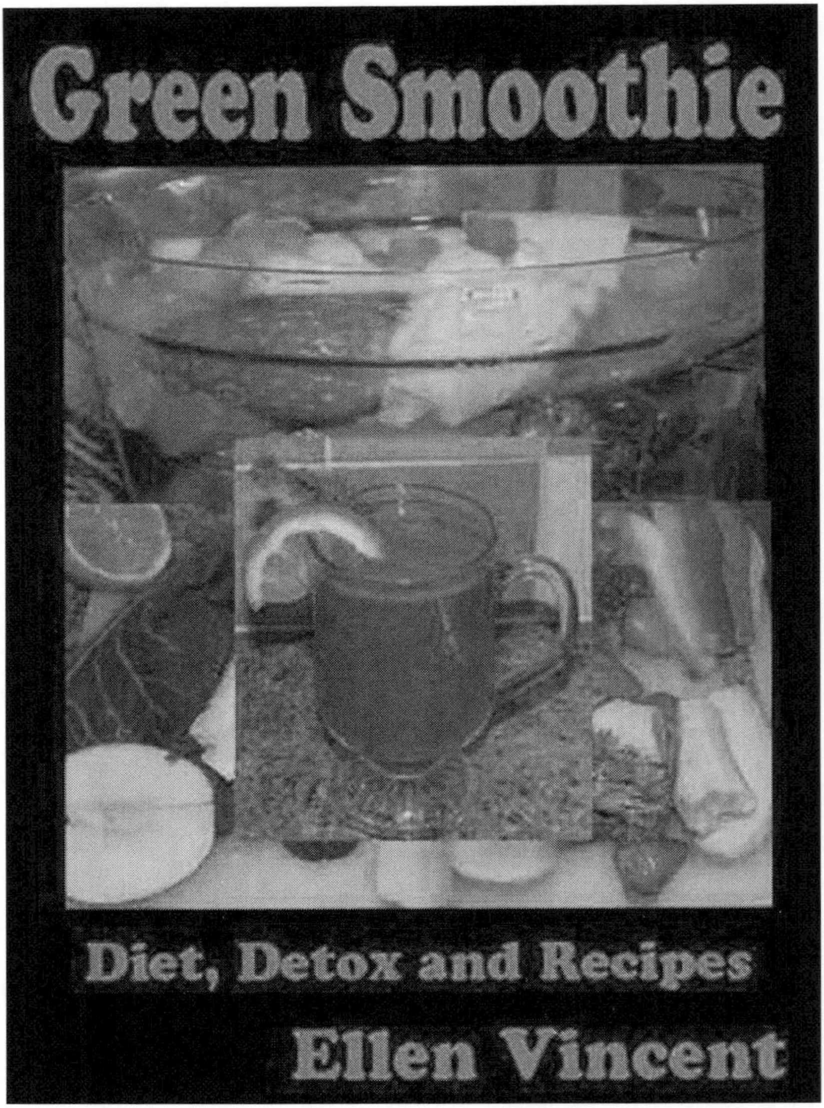

Green smoothies are very popular when it comes to dieting, detoxifying and giving the human body the nutrients that it needs in order to work at the peak of performance. This book explains the many ways that green smoothies can help your body and improve your health and life in general. There are plenty of tips on producing and tailoring green smoothies for your individual needs and there are over 100 exciting recipe ideas included in the book.

Green smoothies give you all of your nutrients the way that nature intended. This means that they are all in their raw form without chemicals, additives and processing. In basic terms you get more out your food when it is consumed in this way. This is because raw food contains more vital nutrients such as vitamins, antioxidants and amino acids. These are so good for your body that people who start eating them can experience a natural high as they are rapidly used up and turned into valuable materials. This means that green smoothies make you feel good as well as doing good.

Green smoothies are a valuable tool when it comes to dieting and losing weight. Due to the fact that they can make you feel fuller for longer they can help you to rapidly lose weight. They can also be the answer to the dieting plateau that many people reach on a normal low calorie diet. There are many other ways that green smoothies can enhance a diet or help in losing weight.

Green Smoothies could be your body's answer to those niggling health problems that can make life a misery. Modern life itself can have a bad effect on the human body and that includes the food that we eat. In seems that the further that we get away from nature, the more problems that we appear to have. If you look back to our ancestors they didn't have supermarkets and chemical additives to preserve and enhance the flavours and appearance of the foods they ate. You have to ask yourself how much damage all of these chemical additives cause? In addition to this even cooking foods causes chemical changes to happen to food and this can result in substances forming which can be bad for us and can even cause certain cancers.

If you feel like life is getting on top of you after too many 'little indulgencies' then green smoothies can be used as a way of detoxifying the body and rapidly returning it to normality.

Green Smoothie provides you with all of the information that you need to get your body working as nature intended. Get the book and join in this exciting new world of health.

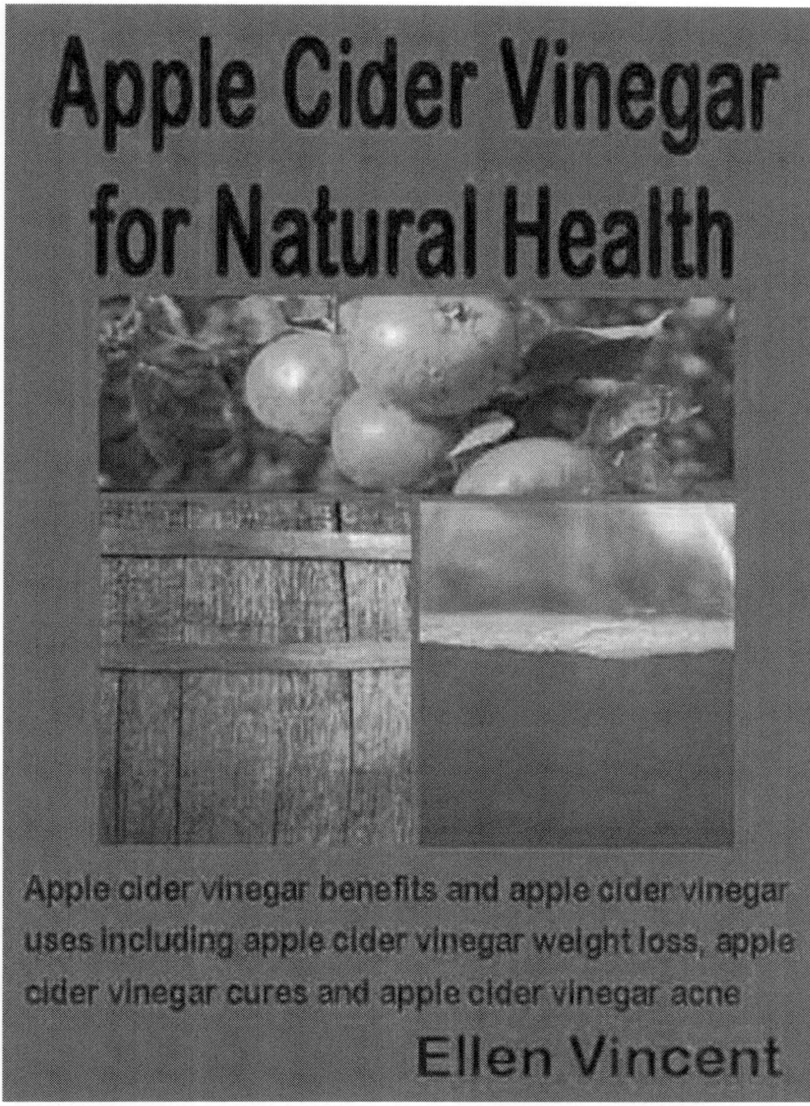

Apple cider vinegar for natural health is all about how you can use this wonderful natural health tonic to improve your life. Apple cider vinegar has been used for centuries to treat a whole host of illnesses and conditions. These cures and remedies have become part of our folklore, but that doesn't mean that we shouldn't take them seriously. Apple cider vinegar contains many health giving substances such as vitamins, minerals, antioxidants, bioflavenoids and of course the main ingredient of acetic acid. All of these things can help our bodies to work to the peak of performance and shrug off some of those day to day conditions that get us down. You can drink apple cider vinegar or apply it directly to the skin or hair. Either way you are getting the benefit of all of these super nutrients. Some books on apple cider vinegar are written by the people who are then trying to sell the vinegar to you. I am not involved in selling these products at all. My main interest comes from my scientific and educational background together with the fact that I use apple cider vinegar myself on many occasions during my day to day life. I am a real fan and take a daily tonic to ward off illness. I also use it on my skin and hair to great effect. I am so impressed with the results that I get with apple cider vinegar that I felt compelled to research it further and then write this book. I have never come across one single substance with so many uses before, and the results can often be stunning. So, take while and look at the information in the book and then try apple cider vinegar for yourself. Pretty soon you could become a real fan too!

This version 2 of the book contains extra information, and in particular details about how to use apple cider vinegar in your daily cooking. There are plenty of recipes and cookery ideas that you can try out for yourself.

4114680R00065

Printed in Germany
by Amazon Distribution
GmbH, Leipzig